Study Guide for

T0195098

Clayton's Basic Pharmacology for Nurses

Study Guide for

Clayton's Basic Pharmacology for Nurses

Nineteenth Edition

Michelle J. Willihnganz, MS, RN, CNE
RCTC Nursing Instructor
Rochester Community and Technical College
Rochester, Minnesota

ELSEVIER

Elsevier
3251 Riverport Lane
St. Louis, Missouri 63043

STUDY GUIDE FOR CLAYTON'S BASIC PHARMACOLOGY FOR NURSES, NINETEENTH EDITION

ISBN: 978-0-323-81259-7

Copyright © 2023 by Elsevier, Inc. All rights reserved.

No part of this publication may be reproduced or transmitted in any form or by any means, electronic or mechanical, including photocopying, recording, or any information storage and retrieval system, without permission in writing from the publisher. Details on how to seek permission, further information about the Publisher's permissions policies and our arrangements with organizations such as the Copyright Clearance Center and the Copyright Licensing Agency, can be found at our website: www.elsevier.com/permissions.

This book and the individual contributions contained in it are protected under copyright by the Publisher (other than as may be noted herein).

Although for mechanical reasons all pages of this publication are perforated, only those pages imprinted with an Elsevier Inc. copyright notice are intended for removal.

Notice

Practitioners and researchers must always rely on their own experience and knowledge in evaluating and using any information, methods, compounds or experiments described herein. Because of rapid advances in the medical sciences, in particular, independent verification of diagnoses and drug dosages should be made. To the fullest extent of the law, no responsibility is assumed by Elsevier, authors, editors or contributors for any injury and/or damage to persons or property as a matter of products liability, negligence or otherwise, or from any use or operation of any methods, products, instructions, or ideas contained in the material herein.

Previous editions copyrighted 2020, 2017, 2013, 2010, 2007, 2004, 2001, and 1997

Content Strategist: Brandi Graham
Content Development Specialist: Rebecca Leenhouts
Publishing Services Manager: Deepthi Unni
Project Manager: Gayathri S
Design Direction: Gopalakrishnan Venkatraman

Printed in India

Last digit is the print number: 9 8 7 6 5 4 3 2

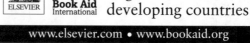

To the Student

This study guide was created to assist you in achieving the objectives of each chapter in *Clayton's Basic Pharmacology for Nurses, Nineteenth Edition*, and establishing a solid base of knowledge in nursing pharmacology. This study guide has been revised to emphasize the chapter objectives with NCLEX-style questions. Completing the questions for each chapter in this guide will help to reinforce the material studied in the textbook and learned in the class. Such reinforcement also helps you to be successful on the NCLEX-PN.

STUDY HINTS FOR ALL STUDENTS

Ask Questions!

There are no stupid questions. If you do not know something or are not sure, you need to find out. Other people may be wondering the same thing but may be too shy to ask. The answer could mean life or death to your patient. That is certainly more important than feeling embarrassed about asking a question.

Chapter Objectives

At the beginning of each chapter in the textbook are objectives that you should have mastered when you finish studying that chapter. Write these objectives in your notebook, leaving a blank space after each. Fill in the answers as you find them while reading the chapter. Review to make sure your answers are correct and complete. Use these answers when you study for tests. This should also be done for separate course objectives that your instructor has listed in your class syllabus.

Key Terms

At the beginning of each chapter in the textbook are key terms that you will encounter as you read the chapter. The key terms are in color the first time they appear significantly in the chapter. Phonetic pronunciations are provided for terms that you might find difficult to pronounce. The goal is to help you if you have limited proficiency in English to develop a greater command of the pronunciation of scientific and nonscientific English terminology. It is hoped that a more general competency in the understanding and use of medical and scientific language may result.

Key Points

Use the key points at the end of each chapter in the textbook to help with review for exams.

Reading Hints

When reading each chapter in the textbook, look at the subject headings to learn what each section is about. Read first for the general meaning. Then reread parts you did not understand. It may help to read those parts aloud. Carefully read the information given in each table and study each figure and its caption.

Concepts

While studying, put difficult concepts into your own words to see if you understand them. Check this understanding with another student or the instructor. Write these in your notebook.

Class Notes

When taking lecture notes in class, leave a large margin on the left side of each notebook page and write only on right-hand pages, leaving all left-hand pages blank. Look over your lecture notes soon after each class, while your memory is fresh. Fill in missing words, complete sentences and ideas, and underline key phrases, definitions, and concepts. At the top of each page, write the topic of that page. In the left margin, write the key word for that part of your notes. On the opposite left-hand page, write a summary or outline that combines material from both the textbook and the lecture. These can be your study notes for review.

Copyright © 2023 by Elsevier, Inc. All rights reserved.

Study Groups

Form a study group with some other students so you can help one another. Practice speaking and reading aloud. Ask questions about material you are not sure about. Work together to find answers.

References for Improving Study Skills

Good study skills are essential for achieving your goals in nursing. Time management, efficient use of study time, and a consistent approach to studying are all beneficial. There are various study methods for reading a textbook and for taking class notes. Some methods that have proven helpful can be found in *Saunders Student Nurse Planner: A Guide to Success in Nursing School.* This book contains helpful information on test taking and preparing for clinical experiences. It includes an example of a "time map" for planning study time and a blank form that you can use to formulate a personal time map.

ADDITIONAL STUDY HINTS FOR ENGLISH AS SECOND-LANGUAGE (ESL) STUDENTS

Vocabulary

If you find a nontechnical word you do not know (e.g., *drowsy*), try to guess its meaning from the sentence (e.g., *With electrolyte imbalance, the patient may feel fatigued and drowsy*). If you are not sure of the meaning, or if it seems particularly important, look it up in the dictionary.

Vocabulary Notebook

Keep a small alphabetized notebook or address book in your pocket or purse. Write down new nontechnical words you read or hear along with their meanings and pronunciations. Write each word under its initial letter so you can find it easily, as in a dictionary. For words you do not know or that have a different meaning in nursing, write down how they are used and sound. Look up their meanings in a dictionary or ask your instructor or first-language buddy. Then write the different meanings or usages that you have found in your book, including the nursing meaning. Continue to add new words as you discover them. For example:

primary	• of most importance; main: *the primary problem or disease*
	• the first one; elementary: *primary school*
secondary	• of less importance; resulting from another problem or disease: *a secondary symptom*
	• the second one: *secondary school (in the United States, high school)*

First-Language Buddy

ESL students should find a first-language buddy – another student who is a native speaker of English and who is willing to answer questions about word meanings, pronunciations, and culture. Maybe your buddy would like to learn about your language and culture also. This could help in their nursing experience as well.

Copyright © 2023 by Elsevier, Inc. All rights reserved.

Contents

Copyright © 2023 by Elsevier, Inc. All rights reserved.

Drug Definitions, Standards, and Information Sources

chapter **1**

Answer Key: Textbook page references are provided as a guide for answering these questions. A complete answer key is provided to your instructor.

MATCHING

Key Term

1. _____ biologic therapies
2. _____ orphan drugs
3. _____ black box warnings
4. _____ pharmacology
5. _____ biosimilars
6. _____ schedules

Definition of a Key Term

a. the study of drugs and their actions on living organisms
b. five classifications of controlled substances
c. an FDA safety concern about a drug after marketing approval
d. medications developed for rare disorders
e. a class of drugs developed to treat autoimmune disorders
f. a biologic product that is close in structure and function to an existing reference product

REVIEW QUESTIONS

Objective: Differentiate among the chemical, generic, and brand names of drugs.

NCLEX item type: multiple choice
Cognitive skill: understanding

7. The nurse recognizes that generic names of drugs are used for which purpose? *(2)*
   1. To describe the exact chemical makeup of the drug.
   2. To provide a simpler way to identify the drug being manufactured.
   3. To market the drug to the public.
   4. To identify illegal drugs.

NCLEX item type: multiple choice
Cognitive skill: comprehension

8. The nurse reviewed the brand names of several drugs which are created for which purpose? *(2)*
   1. To describe the exact chemical makeup of the drug.
   2. To provide a simpler way to identify the drug being manufactured.
   3. To market the drug to the public.
   4. To identify illegal drugs.

NCLEX item type: multiple choice
Cognitive skill: understanding

9. The pharmacist recognizes the chemical constitution of the drug and the exact placement of its molecular groupings and knows it is called what? *(2)*
   1. The chemical name of the drug.
   2. The brand name of the drug.
   3. The generic name of the drug.
   4. The illegal name of the drug.

Objective: Identify the various methods used to classify drugs.

NCLEX item type: multiple response
Cognitive skill: application

10. While studying drugs in school, the nursing student learns that the methods used to classify drugs includes the drug's what? *(Select all that apply.)* *(2)*
    1. Chemical action.
    2. Effect on a body system.
    3. Therapeutic use.
    4. Clinical indication.
    5. Route of administration.

NCLEX item type: multiple response
Cognitive skill: application

11. The nurse was giving examples of drugs that are classified by their physiologic or chemical action to the patient, and included which classifications? *(Select all that apply.)* *(2)*
    1. Anticholinergics
    2. Antacids
    3. Antibiotics
    4. Beta-adrenergic blockers
    5. Antihypertensives

Copyright © 2023 by Elsevier, Inc. All rights reserved.

NCLEX item type: multiple response
Cognitive skill: application

12. The nurse knows that drugs are classified according to body systems, and their effect can involve which systems? *(Select all that apply.)* **(2)**
    1. Cardiovascular system
    2. Respiratory system
    3. Nervous system
    4. Apothecary system
    5. Metric system

NCLEX item type: multiple choice
Cognitive skill: compare

13. The patient asks a nurse what is the difference between biosimilars and generic biologic agents. The nurse responds with which appropriate statement? **(2)**
    1. "As I understand it, the biosimilars are exactly the same as the generic biologic agents, only cheaper."
    2. "The biosimilar agents are manufactured to replace the biologic agents because they are smaller and less complex drugs."
    3. "The biosimilars are close in structure and function to biologics but not identical."
    4. "The biosimilars are more expensive and have predictable reactions compared to biologics."

Objective: Identify sources of drug information available for healthcare providers.

NCLEX item type: multiple response
Cognitive skill: evaluate

14. Which source for drug information would be considered as a reliable database that a nurse can use to get further information on drugs? *(Select all that apply.)* **(3-4)**
    1. *Handbook of Nonprescription Drugs: An Interactive Approach to Self-Care*
    2. *United States Pharmacopeia (USP)/National Formulary (NF)*
    3. Lexi-Comp
    4. Electronic databases such as CINAHL
    5. ePocrates

NCLEX item type: multiple choice
Cognitive skill: understanding

15. A patient has been experiencing adverse effects from a hypertensive medication that was prescribed. The nurse realizes that these adverse effects need to be reported through which program? **(8)**
    1. Watchman program
    2. MedWatch program
    3. PharmWatch program
    4. DrugWatch program

NCLEX item type: multiple choice
Cognitive skill: comprehension

16. A nurse is preparing a scholarly publication on the responses to and adverse effects of heparin. The most efficient and effective means of gathering information for this publication is to use which source? **(3)**
    1. Package inserts from drugs
    2. A consumer health website
    3. Wikipedia
    4. CINAHL database

NCLEX item type: multiple response
Cognitive skill: application

17. As a healthcare professional, it is important that the nurse determine the most accurate and up-to-date Internet information available for drugs that includes which Internet sites? *(Select all that apply.)* **(3)**
    1. ePocrates
    2. DailyMed
    3. Yahoo
    4. Lexicomp
    5. UpToDate

Objective: Discuss the difference between prescription and nonprescription drugs.

NCLEX item type: multiple choice
Cognitive skill: compare

18. The nurse knows that the difference between prescription and nonprescription drugs is that prescription drugs are considered what? **(2)**
    1. To be generally cheaper than nonprescription drugs.
    2. They need to be obtained through a licensed healthcare provider.
    3. Identified using the brand name and nonprescription drugs use the generic name.
    4. That they do not have any serious side effects.

NCLEX item type: multiple choice
Cognitive skill: compare

19. A patient asks the nurse what is the difference between prescription and nonprescription drugs. What is the best response by the nurse? **(2)**
    1. "The difference between the two classifications is really complicated and you just need to follow your healthcare provider's advice."
    2. "Any store that has medications on the shelves indicates that you can purchase them without a prescription."
    3. "The difference between these two types of drugs is that one is the brand name and the other is the generic name."
    4. "Nonprescription drugs do not need to be approved by the FDA and prescription drugs do."

Copyright © 2023 by Elsevier, Inc. All rights reserved.

NCLEX item type: multiple response
Cognitive skill: application

20. Which healthcare providers are licensed to prescribe drugs? *(Select all that apply.)* *(2)*
    1. Pharmacists
    2. Nurses
    3. Physicians
    4. Dentists
    5. Physician assistant

Objective: Describe the process of developing and bringing new drugs to market.

NCLEX item type: multiple choice
Cognitive skill: comprehension

21. Those patients who participate in "testing in humans" are part of which phase of new drug development? *(6)*
    1. Preclinical research and development stage
    2. Clinical research and development stage
    3. New drug application review
    4. Postmarketing surveillance

NCLEX item type: multiple choice
Cognitive skill: understanding

22. When researching how drugs are developed, the nurse found that the phase of drug development dealing with the therapeutic value and whether the drug appears to be safe in animals is known as what? *(6)*
    1. The preclinical research and development stage
    2. The clinical research and development stage
    3. The new drug application review
    4. The postmarketing surveillance

NCLEX item type: multiple choice
Cognitive skill: comprehension

23. The nurse checked to see if the drug that was ordered had a Black Box Warning which indicates what? *(8)*
    1. The drug is associated with an increased risk of causing serious or life-threatening adverse effects.
    2. That the drug has an extremely high cost.
    3. That the drug will cause the adverse effect of nausea and vomiting.
    4. That the drug has an equally effective alternative drug.

Objective: Differentiate between the Canadian *chemical* name and the *proper* name of a drug.

NCLEX item type: multiple choice
Cognitive skill: compare

24. The nurse is discussing the names of drugs with a patient in Canada, explaining that the difference between the chemical drug name and the proper name is what? *(9)*
    1. That the chemical name identifies the manufacturer.
    2. That the proper name of the drug is also the generic name of the drug.
    3. That the proper name is most meaningful to the patient.
    4. That the chemical name identifies the drug as recreational.

NCLEX item type: multiple choice
Cognitive skill: understanding

25. The nurse is discussing drug names with the Canadian patient and remembered that the *proprietary* name of a Canadian drug refers to the drug's what? *(9)*
    1. Generic name
    2. Manufacturer
    3. Classification
    4. Brand name

NCLEX item type: multiple choice
Cognitive skill: comprehension

26. A nurse is explaining to a Canadian patient what is meant by the generic name of the drug and the proper name. Which statement by the nurse is correct? *(9)*
    1. "I believe the brand name of a drug in Canada is too difficult to pronounce."
    2. "I think that generally, the pharmacist uses one name and the physicians use the other name."
    3. "If I recall, the proper Canadian name is easy to remember."
    4. "I understand that the proper Canadian name is usually the generic name of the drug."

Copyright © 2023 by Elsevier, Inc. All rights reserved.

Basic Principles of Drug Action and Drug Interactions

Answer Key: Textbook page references are provided as a guide for answering these questions. A complete answer key is provided to your instructor.

MATCHING

Match the route of administration on the right with the medication on the left. Routes will be used more than once.

Medications

1. _____ oral acetaminophen (Tylenol)
2. _____ subcutaneous insulin (Aspart)
3. _____ intravenous furosemide (Lasix)
4. _____ albuterol (Ventolin) nebulizer
5. _____ sublingual ondansetron (Zofran)

Route of Administration

a. percutaneous
b. enteral
c. parenteral

REVIEW QUESTIONS

Objective: Identify common drug administration routes.
NCLEX item type: multiple response
Cognitive skill: application
6. The nurse knows that drugs are administered by which three most common routes? *(Select all that apply.)* *(14)*
   1. Enteral
   2. Distribution
   3. Percutaneous
   4. Parenteral
   5. Liberation
NCLEX item type: multiple choice
Cognitive skill: understanding
7. The nurse was preparing medications that are to be given by the enteral route which includes medications given how? *(14)*
   1. Subcutaneously
   2. Orally
   3. Transdermally
   4. Intravenously
NCLEX item type: multiple choice
Cognitive skill: comprehension
8. The nurse is explaining to the patient that the drug insulin given as a subcutaneous injection is best absorbed when? *(14)*
   1. After the patient has eaten a meal
   2. When deposited into the correct tissue
   3. After the peripheral circulation is impaired.
   4. When a lump remains at the site of injection

Objective: Identify the meaning and significance of the term *half-life* when used in relation to drug therapy.
NCLEX item type: multiple choice
Cognitive skill: knowledge
9. The nurse understands that the measure of time required for the elimination of a drug from the body is known as what? *(16)*
   1. Expiration time
   2. Minimum life
   3. Circulation time
   4. Half-life
NCLEX item type: multiple choice
Cognitive skill: comprehension
10. The nurse knows that the drug alprazolam (Xanax) has a half-life of 12 hours, which means that how much drug will be left circulating in the body after 24 hours? *(16)*
    1. 50%
    2. 30%
    3. 25%
    4. 15%

Copyright © 2023 by Elsevier, Inc. All rights reserved.

NCLEX item type: multiple response
Cognitive skill: application
11. The nurse explaining to a nursing student the principle of the half-life of a drug, and emphasized that the half-life of a drug may become considerably longer in patients who have which condition(s)? *(Select all that apply.)* **(16)**
    1. Impaired kidney function
    2. Decreased thyroid function
    3. Impaired immune function
    4. Impaired liver function
    5. Decreased amounts of hemoglobin

Objective: Describe the process of how a drug is metabolized in the body.
NCLEX item type: multiple response
Cognitive skill: ordering
12. List in order the five stages that all drugs go through after they have been administered. **(14)**
    1. _____ Metabolism
    2. _____ Distribution
    3. _____ Excretion
    4. _____ Liberation
    5. _____ Absorption
NCLEX item type: multiple response
Cognitive skill: interpret
13. The nurse knows that certain factors effect how fast drugs are transferred from the site of entry into the body to the circulation, and include what? *(Select all that apply.)* **(15)**
    1. Adequate amounts of fluid (usually water) when given orally
    2. Deposited into the correct tissue when given parenterally
    3. A lump remains at the injection site when given subcutaneously
    4. Reconstituted with the correct diluent recommended by the manufacturer
    5. How fine the droplet particles are for inhaled drugs
NCLEX item type: multiple choice
Cognitive skill: compare
14. The nurse understands that drugs are rapidly dispersed throughout the body when administered by which route? **(15)**
    1. Oral
    2. Subcutaneous
    3. Intravenous
    4. Topical

Objective: Compare and contrast the following terms that are used in relationship to medications: *desired action, common adverse effects, serious adverse effects, allergic reactions,* and *idiosyncratic reactions.*
NCLEX item type: multiple choice
Cognitive skill: comprehension
15. Upon review of drug terms, the nurse knows that the term *desired* drug action means what? **(17)**
    1. The predictable/usual response to the drug
    2. An unusual or idiosyncratic response to a drug
    3. A response capable of inducing cell mutations
    4. The unpredictable/unusual response to the drug
NCLEX item type: multiple choice
Cognitive skill: relate
16. The nurse notices that the patient frequently complains about feeling queasy after taking their morning medications. What is the term for this response? **(17)**
    1. The desired effect
    2. A serious adverse effect
    3. A common adverse effect
    4. An idiosyncratic reaction
NCLEX item type: multiple response
Cognitive skill: application
17. Patients who have allergic reactions from an administered drug typically experience which signs/symptoms? *(Select all that apply.)* **(18)**
    1. Severe itching
    2. Hives
    3. Diarrhea
    4. Respiratory distress
    5. Abdominal pain
NCLEX item type: multiple choice
Cognitive skill: interpret
18. A nurse caring for a patient who was hospitalized after developing thrombocytopenia (low platelets) from taking a prescribed medication knows this response is called what? **(17)**
    1. The desired drug effect
    2. An adverse drug effect
    3. An allergic reaction
    4. An idiosyncratic reaction
NCLEX item type: multiple choice
Cognitive skill: explain
19. A patient asked the nurse what the healthcare provider meant by calling his current symptoms *idiosyncratic.* What would be an appropriate response by the nurse? **(18)**
    1. "Your reaction to the medication is really just an allergy."
    2. "The reaction you had to the medication was not what we expected from the drug."
    3. "Your reaction to the drug is typical of what we see from people who have this condition."
    4. "You have had a severe reaction to the medication you are taking and we need to switch your medication."

Copyright © 2023 by Elsevier, Inc. All rights reserved.

Objective: Identify what is meant by a *drug interaction*.

NCLEX item type: multiple response
Cognitive skill: application

20. The nurse knows that drug interactions are said to occur when what happens? *(Select all that apply.)* *(18)*
    1. Interactions occur when one drug increases the action of one or both drugs.
    2. Interactions occur when one drug inhibits the absorption of another.
    3. Interactions occur when drugs are administered 2 hours apart.
    4. Interactions occur when the effectiveness of one drug or both drugs is decreased.
    5. Interactions occur when one drug causes another drug to become displaced from a binding site.

NCLEX item type: multiple choice
Cognitive skill: comprehension

21. The nurse knows that a drug is considered pharmacologically active when what has occurred? *(15)*
    1. When the drug is bound to plasma proteins
    2. When the drug is unbound from plasma proteins
    3. When the drug is distributed evenly throughout the body
    4. When the drug is metabolized by the liver

NCLEX item type: multiple choice
Cognitive skill: comprehension

22. What resources can the nurse use to aid in determining when a drug interaction will occur? *(Select all that apply.)* *(19)*
    1. Consult with the pharmacist.
    2. Look up possible reactions in drug reference books.
    3. Ask the patient when they expect the drugs to interact.
    4. Memorize all possible drug interactions.
    5. Administer each drug several hours apart to ensure nothing happens.

Objective: Differentiate among the terms *additive effect, synergistic effect, antagonistic effect, displacement, interference,* and *incompatibility*.

NCLEX item type: multiple choice
Cognitive skill: understanding

23. The nurse knows that the term for when a combination of two drugs provides a greater effect than the sum of the effect of each drug given alone is called what? *(19)*
    1. Additive effect
    2. Antagonistic effect
    3. Synergistic effect
    4. Displacement effect

NCLEX item type: multiple choice
Cognitive skill: knowledge

24. The nurse knows that the term for the effect of one drug interfering with the effect of another drug is called what? *(19)*
    1. Additive effect
    2. Synergistic effect
    3. Antagonistic effect
    4. Displacement effect

NCLEX item type: multiple choice
Cognitive skill: contrast

25. The nurse knows that the name of a common drug interaction that inhibits the metabolism or excretion of a second drug, thereby causing increased activity of the second drug is called what? *(19)*
    1. Interference
    2. Incompatibility
    3. Antagonistic effect
    4. Additive effect

NCLEX item type: multiple choice
Cognitive skill: interpret

26. The nurse knows that the term for when two drugs that have similar action are taken for an increased effect is called what? *(19)*
    1. Antagonistic effect
    2. Displacement effect
    3. Synergistic effect
    4. Additive effect

NCLEX item type: multiple choice
Cognitive skill: illustrate

27. The nurse knows that the drugs ampicillin and gentamicin are said to be incompatible because they cause what effect? *(19)*
    1. The ampicillin displaces gentamicin from protein-binding sites.
    2. The ampicillin inactivates gentamicin.
    3. The ampicillin inhibits the excretion of gentamicin.
    4. The ampicillin induces enzymes to metabolize gentamicin.

NCLEX item type: multiple choice
Cognitive skill: compare

28. The nurse knows the term *displacement* refers to the drug-drug interaction that causes the first drug to have what effect on the second drug? *(19)*
    1. The first drug inhibits the metabolism of the second drug.
    2. The first drug becomes unbound by the second drug, increasing its effect.
    3. The first drug increases the effect of the second drug.
    4. The first drug decreases the half-life of the second drug.

Copyright © 2023 by Elsevier, Inc. All rights reserved.

Objective: Identify one way in which alternatives in metabolism create drug interactions.

NCLEX item type: multiple choice
Cognitive skill: comprehension

29. The nurse knows that when the enzymes that metabolize drugs are inhibited, then what occurs? *(19)*
    1. There is an increase in drug interactions.
    2. There are more incompatibility issues.
    3. There is an increase in protein-bound drugs.
    4. There is a decrease in absorption rates.

NCLEX item type: multiple choice
Cognitive skill: understands

30. The nurse knows that when the metabolism of a drug is inhibited, then serum drug levels increase and may lead to what effect? *(19)*
    1. Increased displacement
    2. Increased bound drugs
    3. Accumulation and toxicity
    4. Drug incompatibility

NCLEX item type: multiple choice
Cognitive skill: compare

31. What does the nurse expect to see happen when a drug such as rifampin, which binds to an enzyme that increases the metabolism of a second drug? *(19)*
    1. The second drug will generally be decreased
    2. The second drug will generally be increased
    3. The second drug will remain at the same dose
    4. The second drug will have to be discontinued

Copyright © 2023 by Elsevier, Inc. All rights reserved.

Drug Action Across the Life Span

3

Answer Key: Textbook page references are provided as a guide for answering these questions. A complete answer key is provided to your instructor.

MATCHING
Match the correct definition of a drug action with the key term.

Key Term

1. _____ placebo
2. _____ tolerance
3. _____ polypharmacy
4. _____ protein binding
5. _____ teratogens

Definition of a Drug Action

a. the use of multiple drugs for chronic illness that increases risk of drug interactions
b. drugs that cause birth defects
c. how drugs are circulated in the blood
d. a drug form that has no active ingredients
e. when a person needs a higher dose to produce the same effect

REVIEW QUESTIONS

Objective: Explain the impact of the placebo effect and nocebo effect.
NCLEX item type: multiple choice
Cognitive skill: comprehension
6. The nurse is explaining to a patient who is entering into a research study that the patient may actually get a placebo. Which statement by the patient indicates an understanding of the placebo effect? *(23)*
    1. "I will get the drug that they are testing for my condition."
    2. "I could possibly get a pill that will have a negative effect on my condition."
    3. "The placebo is a drug that has no active ingredients."
    4. "The placebo will have the same effect as the real drug."

NCLEX item type: multiple response
Cognitive skill: application
7. The nurse is explaining to the patient the difference between the placebo effect and the nocebo effect. Which statement by the nurse will be included in the discussion? *(Select all that apply.)* *(23)*
    1. "The nocebo effect occurs because the patient has negative expectations about the therapy."
    2. "The placebo effect occurs because the patient has negative expectations about the therapy."
    3. "The nocebo effect occurs because the patient has positive expectations about the therapy."
    4. "The placebo effect occurs because the patient has positive expectations about the therapy."
    5. "The nocebo effect occurs because the patient has no particular expectations about the therapy."

NCLEX item type: multiple choice
Cognitive skill: understanding
8. The attitudes and expectations of the patient regarding the treatment of their condition play a major role in a patient's response to therapy. What does the nurse understand this to mean? *(23)*
    1. That patients with chronic silent conditions such as hypertension are more likely to adhere to the prescribed therapy.
    2. That patients with conditions such as arthritis are least likely to adhere to the therapy prescribed.
    3. That patients with conditions that have rapid consequences if therapy is not followed are more likely to adhere to the prescribed therapy.
    4. That patients who had previous negative experiences are more likely to adhere to the prescribed therapy.

Objective: Identify the importance of drug dependence and drug accumulation.
NCLEX item type: multiple choice
Cognitive skill: comprehension
9. The nurse realizes that drug dependence occurs most often in patients when? *(24)*
    1. When patients are unable to swallow drugs.
    2. When patients have indicated they have adequate pain relief from opioids.
    3. When patients are considered incompetent to make any medical decisions.
    4. When patients develop withdrawal symptoms if the drug is discontinued.
NCLEX item type: multiple choice
Cognitive skill: evaluation
10. What patient action could cause the nurse to suspect that the patient has become dependent on the drug oxycodone? *(24)*
    1. The patient is asking for pain medicine more frequently than prescribed.
    2. The patient has become groggy and hard to arouse about an hour after his dose.
    3. The patient is indicating that there is adequate pain relief with the dose.
    4. The patient is worried about becoming addicted to oxycodone and therefore will not take it.
NCLEX item type: multiple choice
Cognitive skill: understanding
11. The nurse recognizes that when a patient becomes groggy and hard to arouse after receiving a dose of morphine, the patient may be experiencing which drug effect? *(24)*
    1. Dependence
    2. Tolerance
    3. Accumulation
    4. Withdrawal

Objective: Discuss the effects of age on drug absorption, distribution, metabolism, and excretion.
NCLEX item type: multiple choice
Cognitive skill: comprehension
12. In relation to drugs and the aging process, the nurse knows which is true? *(26-27)*
    1. Drugs have the same rate of absorption, distribution, metabolism, and excretion as people age.
    2. Drugs will have the same rate of absorption as people age, but their excretion will be affected by changes in the kidneys.
    3. The liver will increase its ability to metabolize drugs as people age.
    4. Pathologic conditions may alter the rate of drug absorption, distribution, metabolism, and excretion.
NCLEX item type: multiple choice
Cognitive skill: understanding
13. When administering drugs to children, what is important for the nurse to remember? *(30)*
    1. Oral tablets are the easiest dose form to administer to children.
    2. Subcutaneous injections will be the most dangerous drug route to administer to children.
    3. Transdermal drug doses are the most difficult route of administration for children.
    4. Liquid medications are the easiest dose form to administer to children.
NCLEX item type: multiple choice
Cognitive skill: comprehension
14. Crushing medications is often done for ease of administration to older adults, and is considered safe when giving which form of medication? *(31)*
    1. Enteric-coated tablets
    2. Sublingual tablets
    3. Tablet and capsule forms
    4. Timed-release tablets

Objective: Explain the gender-specific considerations of drug absorption, distribution, metabolism, and excretion.
NCLEX item type: multiple response
Cognitive skill: application
15. Drug absorption is influenced by which difference between men and women? *(Select all that apply.)* *(25)*
    1. The difference in the enzyme alcohol dehydrogenase.
    2. The difference in gastric emptying time.
    3. The different enzyme activity (cytochrome P450) between men and women.
    4. The difference in saliva production.
    5. The difference in gastric pH.

Copyright © 2023 by Elsevier, Inc. All rights reserved.

NCLEX item type: multiple choice
Cognitive skill: comprehension

16. The nurse knows that drug distribution is influenced by which difference between men and women? *(26)*
    1. Quantity of fat tissue.
    2. Protein binding.
    3. Gastric emptying time.
    4. Cardiac output.

NCLEX item type: multiple choice
Cognitive skill: understanding

17. The nurse recognizes that drug metabolism is influenced by which difference between men and women? *(27)*
    1. Hereditary characteristics or genes
    2. Number of active receptor sites
    3. General health
    4. Maturity of the enzyme systems

NCLEX item type: multiple choice
Cognitive skill: comprehension

18. The nurse explains to the patient that drug excretion is influenced by which difference between men and women? *(2)*
    1. Renal tubule function
    2. Exhalation of the drug from the lungs
    3. Fat distribution in the body
    4. GI tract motility

Objective: Describe where a nurse will find new information about use of drugs during pregnancy and lactation.

NCLEX item type: multiple choiceCognitive skill: understanding

19. The new rules instituted by the FDA address the use of drugs during pregnancy and breastfeeding. What does the nurse understand about these rules? *(33-34)*
    1. New labeling went into effect for drugs approved since 2001.
    2. New drugs need to be formatted differently for use during pregnancy.
    3. New studies need to be done on drugs known to be teratogenic.
    4. New categories are used for drugs that are approved in pregnancy.

NCLEX item type: multiple response
Cognitive skill: application

20. A new nurse was talking with a seasoned nurse about changes in drug labeling, and the seasoned nurse mentioned that the pregnancy categories have changed. The nurse suggested the new nurse look up the new information on which websites? *(Select all that apply.) (33-34)*
    1. e-Pocrates
    2. Lexicomp
    3. LactMed
    4. HealthNet
    5. DART

NCLEX item type: multiple choice
Cognitive skill: understanding

21. Which online resource for healthcare providers does the nurse use that includes information on drugs during pregnancy and lactation? *(34)*
    1. DailyMed
    2. NANDA
    3. DART
    4. MedMD

Objective: Discuss the impact of pregnancy and breastfeeding on drug absorption, distribution, metabolism, and excretion.

NCLEX item type: multiple choice
Cognitive skill: evaluate

22. The nurse knows that a nursing mother has been taking paroxetine (Paxil) and has explained to her that taking this drug will have what effect? *(34)*
    1. "Paxil will interfere with the metabolism of a nursing infant."
    2. "Paxil is associated with significant effects on nursing infants."
    3. "Paxil has an unknown effect, but may be of concern for a nursing infant."
    4. "Paxil is reported to have adverse effects on nursing infants."

NCLEX item type: multiple choice
Cognitive skill: comprehension

23. The nurse explained to an expectant mother medications that are safe to take during pregnancy and while breastfeeding include which category? *(33)*
    1. Herbal products
    2. Those labeled by the FDA as safe
    3. Those known to be teratogenic
    4. Nonprescription medications only

NCLEX item type: multiple choice
Cognitive skill: compare

24. The nurse applies which general principle to pregnant women with regard to drug therapy? *(34)*
    1. No drugs are safe during pregnancy.
    2. All drugs are safe during pregnancy.
    3. Only drugs that have been approved by the FDA are safe during pregnancy.
    4. All herbal products have been determined as safe during pregnancy.

Objective: Discuss the role of genetics and its influence on drug action.

NCLEX item type: multiple response
Cognitive skill: application

25. The nurse reviewed the characteristics or traits that people get from their ancestors and they include which characteristics? *(Select all that apply.) (35)*
    1. Hair color
    2. Eye color
    3. Food preferences
    4. Skin pigmentation
    5. Parenting style

Copyright © 2023 by Elsevier, Inc. All rights reserved.

NCLEX item type: multiple choice
Cognitive skill: comprehension

26. The nurse explained to a patient why the Human Genome Project is important for biomedical research. Which statement by the nurse is correct? *(35)*
    1. "The genome project is important because it will help predict when a person will get sick."
    2. "The genome project will help researchers study the side effect profiles of different medications."
    3. "The genome project is important because it can now determine what causes cancer."
    4. "The genome project determines which chromosome was inherited from the mother and which from the father."

NCLEX item type: multiple choice
Cognitive skill: evaluate

27. The nurse asked the pharmacist why genetic polymorphisms are important in pharmacology. Which statement by the pharmacist is correct? *(35)*
    1. "Polymorphisms are important because they eliminate drug interactions or drug toxicity."
    2. "Polymorphisms are important because they will impact drug metabolism and excretion."
    3. "Polymorphisms are important because they tend to become teratogenic."
    4. "Polymorphisms are important because they decrease the need for drugs."

Copyright © 2023 by Elsevier, Inc. All rights reserved.

The Nursing Process and Pharmacology

Answer Key: Textbook page references are provided as a guide for answering these questions. A complete answer key is provided to your instructor.

MATCHING

Match the correct definition with the key term

Key Terms

1. _____ nursing process
2. _____ outcome statements
3. _____ defining characteristics
4. _____ core measures
5. _____ focused assessments
6. _____ therapeutic intent
7. _____ tertiary sources

Definition of Key Terms

a. measures track to determine how often hospitals use recommended practice standards
b. information that provides an accurate depiction of the characteristics of a disease
c. the foundation for the clinical practice of nursing
d. why the drug was prescribed and what symptoms will be relieved
e. starts with an action word and need to be SMART
f. signs and symptoms related to a particular patient problem
g. collecting data specific to a patient that validates a suggested problem

REVIEW QUESTIONS

Objective: Discuss the components and purpose of the nursing process.
NCLEX item type: multiple choice
Cognitive skill: understanding
8. Nurses use the nursing process in their work to be able to do what? *(38)*
   1. Build a framework for consistent nursing actions
   2. Assign nursing staff to patients
   3. Standardize the language nurses use to analyze nursing car
   4. Solve problems in nursing systematically
NCLEX item type: multiple choice
Cognitive skill: understanding
9. An important aspect of the nursing process that the nurse uses is based on which approach? *(38)*
   1. Intuitive
   2. systematic
   3. comprehensive
   4. Analytic

NCLEX item type: multiple response
Cognitive skill: ordering
10. List in order the steps used in the nursing process. *(38)*
    1. _____ Nursing diagnosis
    2. _____ Evaluation
    3. _____ Assessment
    4. _____ Planning
    5. _____ Implementation
NCLEX item type: multiple choice
Cognitive skill: understanding
11. The nurse needs to consider the patient's psycho-social and cultural needs during which step of the nursing process? *(40)*
    1. Assessment
    2. Planning
    3. Nursing diagnosis
    4. Implementation

Copyright © 2023 by Elsevier, Inc. All rights reserved.

NCLEX item type: multiple choice
Cognitive skill: comprehension
12. The nurse uses which step of the nursing process to detect any potential complications? *(40)*
    1. Assessment
    2. Planning
    3. Nursing diagnosis
    4. Implementation

Objective: Explain what the nurse does to collect patient information during an assessment.
NCLEX item type: multiple response
Cognitive skill: application
13. Nurses perform the task of patient assessment to determine what? *(Select all that apply.) (39)*
    1. The patient's response to treatments
    2. Any adverse effects of medications
    3. The status of their discharge plans
    4. If the medical diagnosis is correct
    5. If the patient has any risk factors
NCLEX item type: multiple response
Cognitive skill: analyze
14. The initial assessment is performed on a patient to identify patient problems based on defining characteristics, as well as to identify what else? *(Select all that apply.) (39-40)*
    1. Any risk factors that predispose the patient to developing problems
    2. The patient's response to their disease process
    3. Any adverse effects of medications
    4. When the patient needs assistance to get up in the chair
    5. What to prescribe for treatment for various disease processes
NCLEX item type: multiple response
Cognitive skill: application
15. Important healthcare information that the nurse gathers during the assessment of a patient includes which components? *(Select all that apply.) (39)*
    1. Vital signs
    2. Lung sounds
    3. Mobility level
    4. Discharge plans
    5. Family support
NCLEX item type: multiple choice
Cognitive skill: comprehension
16. The nurse needs to assess the patient in the hospital for therapeutic effects, side effects, and potential drug interactions during which time? *(39)*
    1. Throughout the hospitalization
    2. When the patient has visitors
    3. When the patient requests a PRN medication
    4. While monitoring vital signs

Objective: Discuss how nursing diagnosis statements are written.
NCLEX item type: multiple choice
Cognitive skill: understanding
17. What does NANDA stand for when referring to nursing diagnoses? *(41)*
    1. Not All Nursing Diagnosis Association
    2. Natural Accented Northern Diagnosis Adaptable
    3. Nursing Accountable Nursing Diagnosis Authority
    4. North American Nursing Diagnosis Association
NCLEX item type: multiple choice
Cognitive skill: understanding
18. When writing the outcome statement for medication therapy, the nurse will describe the expected outcomes from the prescribed medications based on what? *(41)*
    1. The etiology and contributing factors involved
    2. The patient's laboratory test results
    3. The recommended routes of the medications
    4. The noted improvement of the symptoms present.
NCLEX item type: multiple choice
Cognitive skill: understanding
19. The nurse analyzes the data collected from the patient assessment to identify signs and symptoms that will be addressed under the nursing diagnosis, known as what? *(41)*
    1. Therapeutic intent
    2. Defining characteristics
    3. Measurable outcomes
    4. Contributing factors

Objective: Differentiate between a nursing diagnosis and a medical diagnosis.
NCLEX item type: multiple choice
Cognitive skill: compare
20. Which two types of nursing diagnoses apply to all types of medication therapies? *(41)*
    1. Insufficient knowledge and Insufficient diversional activity
    2. Noncooperation and Insufficient knowledge
    3. Risky health behavior and Noncooperation
    4. Insufficient knowledge and Insufficient family processes
NCLEX item type: multiple choice
Cognitive skill: contrast
21. How do nursing diagnoses differ from medical diagnoses? *(41)*
    1. The medical diagnosis identifies defining characteristics.
    2. The nursing diagnosis identifies alterations in structure and function.
    3. The medical diagnosis identifies alterations in structure and function.
    4. The nursing diagnosis identifies a disease or disorder that impairs function.

Copyright © 2023 by Elsevier, Inc. All rights reserved.

NCLEX item type: multiple choice
Cognitive skill: compare

22. The nurse reviews the three components of the nursing diagnosis and knows they include which ones? *(41)*
    1. Defining characteristics, identified disease processes, and contributing factors
    2. Alterations in function, NANDA-approved label, and identified disease process
    3. Defining characteristics, contributing factors, and etiology of the disorder
    4. NANDA-approved label, defining characteristics, and contributing factors

Objective: Discuss how evidence-based practice is used in planning nursing care.

NCLEX item type: multiple choice
Cognitive skill: comprehension

23. When nurses use evidence-based practice changes for planning nursing care, they are incorporating what factor into the nursing process? *(42)*
    1. Traditional expectations
    2. Trial and error
    3. Pilot studies
    4. Validated research

NCLEX item type: multiple choice
Cognitive skill: comprehension

24. The goal of evidence-based practice is to improve patient outcomes by having the nurse use what? *(42)*
    1. Various treatments for medical conditions
    2. Best practices that evolved from research
    3. The patient's clinical presentation
    4. Prescriptive recommendations of healthcare providers

NCLEX item type: multiple response
Cognitive skill: application

25. Which four phases does the nurse include in the process used for planning patient interventions? *(Select all that apply.)* *(41)*
    1. The nurse sets priorities.
    2. The nurse develops measurable goals.
    3. The nurse identifies "related to" factors.
    4. The nurse formulates nursing interventions.
    5. The nurse formulates therapeutic outcomes.

Objective: Differentiate between nursing interventions and outcome statements.

NCLEX item type: multiple choice
Cognitive skill: compare

26. Nursing interventions identify specific nursing actions, while measurable outcome statements identify specific what? *(41)*
    1. Priority settings
    2. Patient behaviors
    3. Changes in patient care needs
    4. Patient responses

NCLEX item type: multiple choice
Cognitive skill: evaluate

27. Why is it important for nurses to include the patient and appropriate significant others in decision-making when formulating therapeutic patient outcomes? *(43)*
    1. Because it will help promote cooperation and compliance by the patient
    2. Because it will help provide patients with a sense of control over their care
    3. Because it will help prepare the patient for evidence-based nursing care
    4. Because it will help promote shorter hospital stays

NCLEX item type: multiple response
Cognitive skill: application

28. How will the nurse identify the therapeutic outcomes of the medications during the planning phase of the nursing process? *(Select all that apply.)* *(43-44)*
    1. By reviewing the drug monograph for common and serious adverse effects
    2. By filling out an insurance claim for reimbursement
    3. By identifying the therapeutic intent of the medications
    4. By educating the patient how to self-administer medications
    5. By identifying the recommended dosage of the medications

Objective: Explain how Maslow's hierarchy of needs is used to prioritize patient needs.

NCLEX item type: multiple choice
Cognitive skill: understanding

29. When is Maslow's hierarchy of human needs used by nurses in the planning phase of the nursing process? *(42)*
    1. When setting priorities
    2. When developing measurable goals
    3. When formulating therapeutic outcomes
    4. When identifying "related to" factors

NCLEX item type: multiple response
Cognitive skill: application

30. The nurse knows that Maslow's hierarchy of needs include which levels? *(Select all that apply.)* *(42)*
    1. Self-actualization
    2. Safety
    3. Belonging
    4. Physiologic
    5. Priority

NCLEX item type: multiple choice
Cognitive skill: comprehension

31. Which level of Maslow's hierarchy would the nurse use as a priority when planning nursing care? *(42)*
    1. Safety needs
    2. Belonging needs
    3. Self-esteem needs
    4. Physiologic needs

Copyright © 2023 by Elsevier, Inc. All rights reserved.

Objective: Compare and contrast the differences among dependent, interdependent, and independent nursing actions.

NCLEX item type: multiple choice
Cognitive skill: interpret

32. The nurse is performing a *dependent* nursing action in which scenario? *(44)*
    1. The patient is being monitored for the effects of the medication given at 8 AM.
    2. The patient is being educated on her 8 AM medication by the nurse.
    3. The patient is given her 8 AM medication by the nurse.
    4. The patient is verbalizing that she understands the reasons for the medications she received at 8 AM.

NCLEX item type: multiple choice
Cognitive skill: illustrate

33. The nurse is performing an *interdependent* nursing action in which scenario? *(44)*
    1. The nurse is calling the healthcare provider for pain medication prescriptions.
    2. The nurse is assisting the physical therapist with exercises for the patient.
    3. The nurse is assessing the patient for bowel sounds after surgery.
    4. The nurse is educating the patient in the use of incentive spirometer.

NCLEX item type: multiple response
Cognitive skill: application

34. The nurse is performing an *independent* nursing action in which scenarios? *(Select all that apply.)* *(44)*
    1. The patient is being monitored for the effects of the medication given at 8 AM.
    2. The nurse is calling the provider for pain medication prescriptions.
    3. The nurse is educating the patient in the use of the incentive spirometer.
    4. The nurse is assessing the patient for bowel sounds after surgery.
    5. The nurse is consulting with dietary services for patient preference for meals.

Objective: Discuss how the nursing process applies to pharmacology.

NCLEX item type: multiple response
Cognitive skill: application

35. What are the sources that the nurse uses to obtain a medication history? *(Select all that apply.)* *(45)*
    1. Objective data (observed by the nurse)
    2. Other healthcare professionals
    3. Subjective data (provided by the patient)
    4. Drug monographs
    5. The electronic medical record

NCLEX item type: multiple response
Cognitive skill: explain

36. When discussing the medication history with a patient, the nurse will ask the patient to identify current medications and drug allergies, as well as what other important factor(s)? *(Select all that apply.)* *(45)*
    1. Any diagnostic tests done
    2. Any over-the-counter medications used
    3. Any food allergies
    4. Any herbal products used
    5. Any street drugs used

NCLEX item type: multiple choice
Cognitive skill: interpret

37. The nurse can use primary, secondary, and tertiary sources to gain information to complete the medication history. When the nurse obtains vital signs to use as monitoring parameters later, it is considered which source of information? *(45)*
    1. A secondary source of information
    2. A tertiary source of information
    3. A primary source of subjective data
    4. A primary source of objective data

NCLEX item type: multiple choice
Cognitive skill: comprehension

38. The medication history that the nurse records includes which important facts to note? *(45)*
    1. Current medications being taken by the patient and drug allergies
    2. Past medications that are no longer being used and drug allergies
    3. Medications that are prescription-based and drug allergies
    4. Over-the-counter medications and drug allergies

Copyright © 2023 by Elsevier, Inc. All rights reserved.

Patient Education to Promote Health

Answer Key: Textbook page references are provided as a guide for answering these questions. A complete answer key is provided to your instructor.

MATCHING
Match the learning domain on the right with the patient education objective on the left. Domains may be used more than once.

Patient Education Objective

1. _____ demonstrating correct self-administration of insulin

2. _____ sorts the medication into the pill container properly

3. _____ requesting more information on adverse effects of a new medication

4. _____ appears worried regarding

5. _____ discussing healthcare changes that will occur when discharged, like needing an aide

6. _____ verbalizing the medications needed for pain relief after surgery

Learning Domain

a. cognitive domain
b. affective domain
c. psychomotor domain

REVIEW QUESTIONS

Objective: Differentiate among cognitive, affective, and psychomotor learning domains.
NCLEX item type: multiple choice
Cognitive skill: understanding
7. When the nurse asks the patient to perform a return demonstration of a skill such as injecting insulin or performing a dressing change, the patient is exercising which domain of learning? *(51)*
   1. Affective
   2. Psychomotor
   3. Cognitive
   4. Psychologic

NCLEX item type: multiple choice
Cognitive skill: compare
8. The nurse explains to the patient that the *affective* domain of learning refers to what? *(50)*
   1. The thinking portion of the learning process
   2. Learning a new procedure or skill
   3. Feelings, beliefs, and values that the patient has
   4. The environment that is conducive to learning

NCLEX item type: multiple choice
Cognitive skill: classify
9. The patient has just been instructed on his home-going medications prior to discharge, and the nurse will validate the information that was given by asking the patient to verbalize his understanding. This involves which domain of learning? *(50)*
   1. Cognitive
   2. Affective
   3. Psychomotor
   4. Psychologic

Objective: Identify the main principles of learning that are applied when teaching a patient, family, or group.
NCLEX item type: multiple choice
Cognitive skill: evaluate
10. When teaching patients and their families, the nurse must recognize the teachable moment when what occurs? *(51)*
   1. The nurse starts to ask questions regarding home-going care.
   2. The nurse has the time and is ready to start teaching the patient.
   3. The patient is gone for a test and the family looks anxious.
   4. The patient starts to ask questions about what to expect when at home.

Copyright © 2023 by Elsevier, Inc. All rights reserved.

NCLEX item type: multiple choice
Cognitive skill: understanding
11. One of the main principles of learning that the nurse incorporates into teaching is that adults learn by what? *(50)*
    1. Rote memorization
    2. Applying new knowledge to previous learning
    3. Listening to the nurse explain everything
    4. Asking questions

NCLEX item type: multiple response
Cognitive skill: application
12. The nurse needs to determine the patient's preferred learning style when educating the patient on continuing care. One way to do this is by using a variety of teaching aids, which may include what examples? *(Select all that apply.)* *(51)*
    1. Pamphlets and charts
    2. Discussing care with the family while the patient is out
    3. DVDs and videos
    4. Smart devices and computer-aided instruction
    5. Filling out the nursing care plan and informing the next shift about it

Objective: Describe the essential elements of patient education in relation to prescribed medications.
NCLEX item type: multiple response
Cognitive skill: evaluation
13. When the nurse is teaching the patient about medications, which important considerations can be implemented? *(Select all that apply.)* *(51)*
    1. Teaching at a time most convenient for the nurse
    2. Determining the patient's readiness to learn
    3. Spacing the content over several short sessions
    4. Organizing the patient education materials
    5. Using repetition to enhance learning

NCLEX item type: multiple choice
Cognitive skill: comprehension
14. During a teaching session, the patient suddenly became tearful and turned away. What would be the best response from the nurse at this time? *(54)*
    1. "Why don't you just read this later, and I can mark you as getting through the material."
    2. "I need to finish this and get it checked off my list, so bear with me."
    3. "I see that you are upset; I can finish this later. Do you want to talk about it?"
    4. "I see that you are not paying attention. Now come on, let's finish this."

NCLEX item type: multiple response
Cognitive skill: analyze
15. When teaching older adults about new medications, what is important for the nurse to remember? *(Select all that apply.)* *(56-57)*
    1. Check the patient for vision or hearing aids
    2. Determine any memory impairment
    3. Evaluate the gross motor ability of the patient
    4. Review the content to be covered rapidly
    5. Lecture the patient about healthy lifestyles

Objective: Describe the nurse's role in fostering patient responsibility for maintaining well-being and for adhering to the therapeutic regimen.
NCLEX item type: multiple response
Cognitive skill: application
16. The nurse understands that when teaching a patient and family about lifestyle changes, it is important to do which of the following? *(Select all that apply.)* *(55-56)*
    1. Tell the patient that they will need to change their lifestyle or else
    2. Keep the content of the information relevant to the patient
    3. Add extra content to further explain points
    4. Remember that learning new ideas may be overwhelming
    5. Keep the patient's wishes in mind

NCLEX item type: multiple choice
Cognitive skill: illustrate
17. What is one important aspect of the nurse's role in discussing the patient's medications and adhering to a particular medication regimen? *(57)*
    1. To adopt a slower pace for teaching younger patients
    2. To dictate to the older adult patient what must be changed
    3. To continue teaching until all content is covered
    4. To repeat the information often, and stop and allow practice

NCLEX item type: multiple response
Cognitive skill: evaluate
18. The nurse needs to involve the patient in cooperative goal-setting when teaching, which will include discussing what with the patient? *(Select all that apply.)* *(57-58)*
    1. What the patient should monitor
    2. Why the prescribed therapy is needed
    3. When to call the healthcare provider
    4. Where to collect and record essential data
    5. How to discontinue or alter their medication regimen

Objective: Identify the types of information that should be discussed with the patient or significant others.
NCLEX item type: multiple response
Cognitive skill: application
19. The nurse is reviewing sources of patient information on the Internet that may be helpful for patients wanting more information after discharge. These sources may include which websites? *(Select all that apply.)* *(56)*
    1. Krames Online
    2. Healthcare institution intranet
    3. Health on the Net Foundation
    4. Medline
    5. CINAHL

Copyright © 2023 by Elsevier, Inc. All rights reserved.

NCLEX item type: multiple choice
Cognitive skill: interpret

20. Nurses who tend to be ethnocentric generally consider patients in light of what? *(55)*
    1. The culture the patient is from
    2. The culture the nurse is from
    3. The hospital the patient is in
    4. The home environment the patient lives in

NCLEX item type: multiple choice
Cognitive skill: relate

21. Reasonable expectations that the nurse should have when discussing new treatment therapies include which factor? *(56-57)*
    1. That the patient will fully understand all instructions
    2. That the patient and family will ask appropriate questions and demonstrate adequate understanding of teaching
    3. That the family will have participated in the teaching because most patients are unable to think clearly while in the hospital
    4. That the patient will need to be taken care of outside of the hospital, since the instructions will never be understood

NCLEX item type: multiple choice
Cognitive skill: evaluate

22. After the nurse finished teaching the patient and asked for teach back, which statement by the patient indicates that further teaching is needed? *(52)*
    1. "I will keep a record of my blood pressure the same time of day to see how my medication is working."
    2. "I know that I will need to call my healthcare provider when I start to feel like I did when I came into the hospital."
    3. "I can take my pills when I feel like it, because they can get so expensive."
    4. "I will let my wife know about these pills because she usually helps me remember to take them."

Copyright © 2023 by Elsevier, Inc. All rights reserved.

Principles of Medication Administration and Medication Safety

chapter
6

Answer Key: Textbook page references are provided as a guide for answering these questions. A complete answer key is provided to your instructor.

MATCHING

Match the rights of drug administration on the right with the nursing action on the left. Rights may be used more than once.

Nursing Action

1. _____ triple-check the drug
2. _____ consult reference book and calculate properly
3. _____ verify the reason for the drug
4. _____ this affects absorption rate
5. _____ check to determine when drug was given last
6. _____ compare exact spelling
7. _____ a major medicolegal consideration
8. _____ ensure two identifiers are used
9. _____ determine appropriate schedule

Seven Rights of Drug Administration

a. right drug
b. right indication
c. right time
d. right dose
e. right patient
f. right route
g. right documentation

REVIEW QUESTIONS

Objective: Identify the legal and ethical considerations for medication administration.

NCLEX item type: multiple choice
Cognitive skill: comprehension

10. The rules and regulations established by the state boards of nursing are in place to ensure what? **(60-61)**
    1. That there are guidelines in place to practice nursing
    2. To restrict access to healthcare
    3. What will be done when an avoidable complication arises
    4. To regulate healthcare facilities

NCLEX item type: multiple response
Cognitive skill: application

11. Policy statements made by nurse practice acts related to medication administration include which examples? *(Select all that apply.)* **(61)**
    1. Educational requirements for those individuals administering medications
    2. Lists of medications that are forbidden to be administered by nurses
    3. Abbreviations approved for use to avoid medication errors
    4. Medications that the nurse can start with IV solutions
    5. When to claim unfamiliarity with any nursing responsibilities

Copyright © 2023 by Elsevier, Inc. All rights reserved.

NCLEX item type: multiple response
Cognitive skill: analyze

12. Prior to any medication administration, the nurse must be able to do what? *(Select all that apply.)* **(61)**
    1. Accurately calculate the drug dose
    2. Document the patient's response to the medication
    3. Explain to the patient the expected actions of the medication
    4. Explain to the patient why the medication is prescribed
    5. Describe the contraindications for the use of the medication

Objective: Compare and contrast the various systems used to dispense medications.

NCLEX item type: multiple response
Cognitive skill: application

13. The nurse knowns that the floor stock system of dispensing medications used in small hospitals has not only the advantage of readily available medications, but also what disadvantage? *(Select all that apply.)* **(67)**
    1. There is increased potential for medication errors.
    2. There is the potential misappropriation of medication by hospital personnel.
    3. There are fewer inpatient prescription orders.
    4. There is a lack of review by a pharmacist for patient prescription accuracy.
    5. There is a need for larger stocks and frequent drug inventories.

NCLEX item type: multiple choice
Cognitive skill: comprehension

14. Which system does the nurse use to dispense medications that provides the advantage of fewer inpatient prescription orders and a minimal return of medications? **(67)**
    1. The unit-dose system
    2. The floor or ward stock system
    3. The individual prescription order system
    4. The computer-controlled dispensing system

NCLEX item type: multiple choice
Cognitive skill: compare

15. The nurse understands that there are advantages of the unit-dose system which include what? **(67-68)**
    1. Returned bottles of unused medications are destroyed.
    2. There is less waste and misappropriation of medications.
    3. A passcode is utilized to access the system prior to removal of medications.
    4. Packaging of medications require counting drugs from multidose packets.

NCLEX item type: multiple choice
Cognitive skill: compare

16. The nurse is using the *pyxis system* which refers to what drug dosage system? **(68)**
    1. Narcotic inventory system
    2. Individual prescription order system
    3. Unit-dose system used primarily in long-term care
    4. Computer-controlled dispensing system

NCLEX item type: multiple choice
Cognitive skill: comprehension

17. The nurse knows that the *ward stock system* refer to what? **(67)**
    1. A narcotic inventory system
    2. An individual prescription order system
    3. A system used in very small hospitals
    4. An electronic medication dispensing system

NCLEX item type: multiple choice
Cognitive skill: interpret

18. The nurse understands that using a computer-controlled dispensing system means what? **(68)**
    1. That there is no need to use standard procedures for medications like the seven rights.
    2. That the verification and transcription of medication prescriptions are built into the system.
    3. The need to account for the narcotic inventory will no longer be necessary.
    4. Documentation of the patient's response to the medication is not needed.

Objective: Identify what a narcotic control system entails.

NCLEX item type: multiple response
Cognitive skill: illustrate

19. When removing narcotics from a narcotic control system, what must the nurse be recording at the time of removal? *(Select all that apply.)* **(69)**
    1. The medications must be passcode-accessible
    2. The name of the patient
    3. The time the medication was removed
    4. The name of the nurse who removed the medication
    5. The time the medication was given to the patient

NCLEX item type: multiple response
Cognitive skill: application

20. A nurse was preparing to administer 3 mg of morphine (a controlled substance) orally to a patient. The medication came in 4 mg/4 mL. What steps must the nurse take when giving this medication? *(Select all that apply.)* **(69)**
    1. Determine the correct amount to give (3 mL).
    2. Ask another nurse to verify the dose and any wasted medication.
    3. Check the time interval since the last dose was given.
    4. Complete the controlled substance inventory.
    5. Complete the documentation after administration.

Copyright © 2023 by Elsevier, Inc. All rights reserved.

NCLEX item type: multiple choice
Cognitive skill: comprehension
21. While checking the narcotics count at the end of a shift, the nurse notes a discrepancy regarding the oral doses of hydromorphone (Dilaudid). What needs to be done next? *(70)*
    1. Security needs to be called.
    2. The nurse manager needs to be notified.
    3. The patients' charts need to be reviewed for proper documentation.
    4. An appropriate interval of time must be observed before any narcotics can be removed.

Objective: Identify common types of medication errors and the actions that can be taken to prevent them.
NCLEX item type: multiple choice
Cognitive skill: relate
22. The nurse is preparing to administer a patient's 8 AM medications and notes that the dose for the drug raloxifene (Evista) is only 20 mg and not 40 mg. What will the nurse need to do next? *(74)*
    1. Verify the dosage with the healthcare provider.
    2. Notify the pharmacy that the drug dose is in error.
    3. Administer the medication and report the error.
    4. Refuse to administer all of the patient's medications until the error is corrected.

NCLEX item type: multiple response
Cognitive skill: application
23. Which type of medication errors could a nurse make when administering a drug? *(Select all that apply.)* *(72)*
    1. Errors of omission (missed dose)
    2. Errors of duplication (extra dose given)
    3. Errors of inventory of the drugs
    4. Errors of formatting the prescription wrong
    5. Errors of wrong time

NCLEX item type: multiple response
Cognitive skill: compare
24. Technology is being used to help nurses and to prevent medication errors by which methods? *(Select all that apply.)* *(72-73)*
    1. Robotics to administer medications to free up nurses
    2. System of automatic delivery of medications
    3. Programs that have computerized provider order entry systems
    4. Smart pumps for controlled administration of controlled medications
    5. Barcoded labeling of medications for administration

NCLEX item type: multiple choice
Cognitive skill: comprehension
25. After administering a dose of the oral antihistamine fexofenadine (Allegra), the nurse noticed the patient had already received a dose 2 hours before. What is this type of error called? *(72)*
    1. A prescribing error
    2. An administration error
    3. A monitoring error
    4. A transcription error

NCLEX item type: multiple choice
Cognitive skill: contrast
26. During the administration of a medication, the patient asks the nurse why the medication has been prescribed. The nurse will respond with which one of the seven rights? *(74-75)*
    1. Right patient
    2. Right route
    3. Right dosage
    4. Right indication

NCLEX item type: multiple response
Cognitive skill: application
27. When preparing to administer a medication to a patient, the nurse is not able to verify that the medication prescription is appropriate. What actions does the nurse take? *(Select all that apply.)* *(74)*
    1. Contacts the healthcare provider who prescribed the drug
    2. Documents the reasons for refusal to administer the drug in accordance with the policies of the agency
    3. Informs the patient about the disagreement with the treatment prescribed
    4. If the prescriber cannot be contacted, notifies the nursing supervisor on duty
    5. Administers the medication because it went through pharmacy, and they would have caught a problem if there was one

Objective: Identify precautions used to ensure the right drug is prepared and given to the right patient.
NCLEX item type: multiple response
Cognitive skill: ordering
28. The nurse was preparing to administer a dose of the antibiotic cefepime. Place the steps in the order that the nurse will follow to ensure the right drug is administered. *(74-77)*
    1. _____ Document the drug.
    2. _____ Triple-check that the drug name and dose are correct prior to administration.
    3. _____ Identify the patient using two patient identifiers.
    4. _____ Administer the medication via the correct route.
    5. _____ Check the prescription.

Copyright © 2023 by Elsevier, Inc. All rights reserved.

NCLEX item type: multiple response
Cognitive skill: application

29. Medication reconciliation is a process designed to reduce medication errors and involves which steps? *(Select all that apply.)* **(73)**
    1. Comparing written blanket prescriptions
    2. Reviewing potential adverse drug events
    3. Developing a list of prescribed medications
    4. Developing a list of current medications being taken by the patient
    5. Comparing the lists of current medications with prescribed ones

NCLEX item type: multiple choice
Cognitive skill: relate

30. What is the most effective method the nurse uses for identifying a pediatric patient for medication administration? **(76)**
    1. Asking the child their name
    2. Asking a family member the child's name
    3. Checking the child's identification bracelet
    4. Checking the room number with the bed the child is in

Objective: Identify the appropriate nursing documentation of medications including the effectiveness of each medication.

NCLEX item type: multiple response
Cognitive skill: application

31. What does the nurse need to document to identify how effective medications are? *(Select all that apply.)* **(77)**
    1. Questions the family asks about home-going medications
    2. Noting any nausea and vomiting after giving oral medications
    3. Monitoring the patient's vital signs
    4. Checking blood sugar after insulin administration
    5. Specific assessments such as lung sounds

NCLEX item type: multiple choice
Cognitive skill: comprehension

32. What does the nurse need to do when determining the therapeutic effectiveness of a medication? **(75)**
    1. Ask the patient to repeat the name of the medication.
    2. Call the healthcare provider to verify each medication prescribed.
    3. Notify the pharmacist of the patient's response.
    4. Document the patient's response and notify the healthcare provider when appropriate.

NCLEX item type: multiple choice
Cognitive skill: explain

33. The nurse gave an antiemetic medication 30 minutes ago and is checking on the patient to determine the effectiveness. Which scenario indicates the medication worked? **(75)**
    1. The patient feels much better and his pain is all gone.
    2. The patient feels a lot less nauseated.
    3. The patient is starting to feel dizzy and lightheaded.
    4. The patient is feeling weaker and getting chills.

Copyright © 2023 by Elsevier, Inc. All rights reserved.

Percutaneous Administration

Answer Key: Textbook page references are provided as a guide for answering these questions. A complete answer key is provided to your instructor.

MATCHING
Match the dose form on the right with the application site on the left. More than one dose form may be used for the application sites.

Application Site

1. _____ ear
2. _____ eye
3. _____ skin
4. _____ mucous membranes
5. _____ buccal cavity

Dose Form

a. powders
b. aqueous solutions
c. transdermal patches
d. creams
e. ointments
f. buccal tablets

REVIEW QUESTIONS

Objective: Identify the equipment needed and the techniques used to apply each of the topical forms of medications to the skin.

NCLEX item type: multiple response
Cognitive skill: application

6. The nurse is aware of the factors affecting the absorption of topical medications which include what factors? *(Select all that apply.) (83)*
   1. The concentration of the medication
   2. The length of time the medication is in contact with the skin
   3. The patient's personal hygiene preferences
   4. The thickness and hydration of the skin
   5. The size and depth of the skin area

NCLEX item type: multiple response
Cognitive skill: application

7. The nurse recognizes the major advantages of the percutaneous route for medication administration and knows they include which factors? *(Select all that apply.) (83)*
   1. This route reduces the spread of infection.
   2. This route decreases systemic adverse effects.
   3. This route improves patient personal hygiene measures.
   4. This route has a long duration of action and reapplication is often not required.
   5. This route allows for limited exposure of the medication to a specific site of application.

NCLEX item type: multiple response
Cognitive skill: application

8. The nurse explains to the patient the different forms of application that are used for the percutaneous route and includes in the discussion which examples? *(Select all that apply.) (83)*
   1. Eyedrops
   2. Nasal sprays
   3. Rectal suppositories
   4. Subcutaneous injections
   5. Inhaled nebulized medications

NCLEX item type: multiple choice
Cognitive skill: comprehension

9. Why is it important for the nurse to wear gloves when applying a topical ointment or transdermal patch? *(84)*
   1. To identify a patient's sensitivity to contact materials
   2. So the correct amount of medication is applied to the patient's skin
   3. So the dose is not contaminated with the nurse's skin cells
   4. To avoid inadvertent absorption of the medication by the nurse through the skin

Copyright © 2023 by Elsevier, Inc. All rights reserved.

NCLEX item type: multiple response
Cognitive skill: ordering
10. List the steps in the order in which the nurse would apply a medicated lotion to a patient. *(84-85)*
    1. _____ Apply lotion firmly but gently by dabbing the surface.
    2. _____ Perform hand hygiene and apply gloves.
    3. _____ Document the application.
    4. _____ Shake the suspension well for a uniform appearance of the lotion.
    5. _____ Clean the area and the equipment used, and make sure that the patient is comfortable.

Objective: Describe the purpose of and the procedure used for performing patch testing.
NCLEX item type: multiple choice
Cognitive skill: comprehension
11. The nurse is performing a patch test and know the purpose is to identify what? *(85)*
    1. When a patient will need an antiemetic
    2. Which antibiotic will be effective against an infection
    3. Which allergen the patient has a specific sensitivity to
    4. Which area of the patient's skin is sensitive to topical ointments

NCLEX item type: multiple choice
Cognitive skill: understanding
12. The nurse is preparing to apply a patch test to a patient, and the patient asks what they need to remember after leaving the clinic. Which response by the nurse would be most appropriate? *(86-87)*
    1. "You will need to call the clinic in 48 hours if you have a reaction."
    2. "You will need to report back to the clinic after a week and we will read the results."
    3. "You will not be able to shower for a week while the patch test is on your back."
    4. "You will need to return to the clinic to have the test read in 48 hours."

NCLEX item type: multiple response
Cognitive skill: compare
13. The nurse identified the common areas for patch testing to the patient. What areas on the body are commonly used for a patch test? *(Select all that apply.) (86)*
    1. Face
    2. Thighs
    3. Back
    4. Neck
    5. Arms

NCLEX item type: multiple response
Cognitive skill: application
14. The nurse reviewed the symbols commonly used for reading reactions to allergen testing. Which are examples that correctly identify a response? *(Select all that apply.) (86)*
    1. ++ (2+) (2- to 3-mm wheal with flare)
    2. ## (2#) (only erythema noted)
    3. – – – (3–) (no wheal response)
    4. ++++ (4+) (> 5-mm wheal)
    5. +++ (3+) (3- to 5-mm wheal with flare)

NCLEX item type: multiple response
Cognitive skill: application
15. The nurse is working in an allergy clinic. What should the nurse consider when administering allergy testing to patients? *(Select all that apply.) (86)*
    1. Documenting "no reaction" at the control site on the patient's chart
    2. Ensuring that emergency equipment is in the immediate area in case of an anaphylactic response
    3. Administering antihistamine and antiinflammatory agents immediately before the test
    4. Positioning the patient so that the surface where the test material is to be applied is horizontal
    5. Cleansing the area where the allergens are to be applied with an alcohol wipe and allowing the area to dry before starting testing

Objective: Identify the equipment needed, the sites and techniques used, and the patient education required when nitroglycerin ointment is prescribed.
NCLEX item type: multiple response
Cognitive skill: ordering
16. List in the correct order the steps the nurse will use to administer nitroglycerin ointment. *(87-88)*
    1. _____ Position patient to expose surface to be used, and remove applicator paper from previous dose.
    2. _____ Apply dose to patient's skin and cover with plastic wrap or tape.
    3. _____ Perform hand hygiene and don gloves.
    4. _____ Gather nitroglycerin ointment, applicator paper, and nonallergenic adhesive tape.
    5. _____ Squeeze proper amount of nitroglycerin ointment onto applicator paper.

NCLEX item type: multiple choice
Cognitive skill: knowledge
17. The nurse is applying a nitroglycerin transdermal disk and expects the disk to be applied how often? *(89)*
    1. Every 12 hours
    2. Every day
    3. Every 7 days
    4. Every 3 days

Copyright © 2023 by Elsevier, Inc. All rights reserved.

NCLEX item type: multiple choice
Cognitive skill: comprehension
18. After applying a nitroglycerin transdermal disk, what should the nurse educate the patient about? *(89-90)*
    1. The number of times the disks can be reused
    2. The documentation needed after application
    3. How and when to apply the disks
    4. To never wear the disks while showering

NCLEX item type: multiple choice
Cognitive skill: interpret
19. The nurse will identify the expected effectiveness of the nitroglycerin ointment when the patient states what has occurred? *(87)*
    1. Itching and a rash with the drug
    2. An increase in angina attacks
    3. Relief from angina attacks
    4. A severe drop in blood pressure and lightheadedness

NCLEX item type: multiple response
Cognitive skill: analyze
20. What should the nurse include in the documentation of the application of nitroglycerin ointment? *(Select all that apply.) (88)*
    1. When any family is present in the room
    2. That essential patient education that was reviewed
    3. The signs and symptoms of adverse drug effects
    4. The date, time, dosage, site, route of administration, and nurse's name
    5. The patient assessments such as blood pressure, pulse, and pain relief

Objective: Identify the equipment needed, the sites and techniques used, and the patient education required when transdermal medication systems are prescribed.

NCLEX item type: multiple response
Cognitive skill: application
21. What does patient education for transdermal medication systems include? *(Select all that apply.) (89-90)*
    1. When to document the administration of the medication
    2. When it is appropriate to take a shower
    3. What to do when the disk becomes loose
    4. When a drug-free period of time is prescribed
    5. When to discontinue using the medication

NCLEX item type: multiple choice
Cognitive skill: comprehension
22. When administering nitroglycerin percutaneously to a patient, what does the nurse do? *(87-88)*
    1. Performs hand hygiene and wears gloves
    2. Applies wax paper over the site of the nitroglycerin ointment to enhance absorption of the drug
    3. Ensures that the drug is on the patient 24 hours a day, 7 days a week to avoid complications
    4. Always places the nitroglycerin ointment over the left chest to provide the most effective route of drug delivery to the heart

NCLEX item type: multiple response
Cognitive skill: application
23. The nurse discussed the common sites used for application of any transdermal medication disks with the patient and includes which areas of the body? *(Select all that apply.) (89)*
    1. Chest
    2. Face
    3. Flank
    4. Upper arms
    5. Axilla

NCLEX item type: multiple choice
Cognitive skill: illustrate
24. The nurse is reviewing a prescription to administer a topical powder to a patient. What should the nurse know prior to administration? *(84)*
    1. The site of application, the indication for the medication, and the expected effects
    2. The site of application, the common adverse effects of the medication, and the family's expectations
    3. The site of application, the indication for the medication, and the patient's usual sleep pattern
    4. The site of application, the patient's bathing preference, and the expected effects

NCLEX item type: multiple response
Cognitive skill: application
25. The nurse will perform proper administration of powdered medications which includes which technique? *(84) (Select all that apply.)*
    1. Applying the powder to wet skin to allow it to "cake" on
    2. Applying the powder over the area, distributing it evenly and smoothing over the area
    3. Shaking the container prior to administration to evenly distribute the medication
    4. Performing hand hygiene before and after administration; gloves are not necessary
    5. Instruct the patient to turn their head to avoid inhaling any powder

NCLEX item type: multiple choice
Cognitive skill: knowledge
26. The nurse understands an important point to consider when administering powdered medication and remembers it involves what? *(84)*
    1. How long the powder needs to stay on
    2. When to wash the powder off
    3. Where to apply the powder
    4. Which medication will wear off faster

Copyright © 2023 by Elsevier, Inc. All rights reserved.

Objective: Describe the dose forms, the sites and equipment used, and the techniques for the administration of medications to the mucous membranes.

NCLEX item type: multiple response
Cognitive skill: ordering

27. List in order the steps the nurse will take to administer eyedrops. *(91)*
    1. _____ Hold the eyelid open and approach the eye from below with the medication dropper.
    2. _____ Discard gloves, perform hand hygiene, and document.
    3. _____ Position the patient so that the back of the head is firmly supported on a pillow and the face is directed toward the ceiling.
    4. _____ Obtain the prescribed bottle or tube of eye medication.
    5. _____ Perform hand hygiene and don gloves.

NCLEX item type: multiple choice
Cognitive skill: comprehension

28. The nurse explained the proper technique to the patient regarding how to administer eyedrops or eye ointment and asks the patient to look in which direction? *(91)*
    1. Down and to the left
    2. Up and over your head
    3. Up and to the right
    4. Down and to the right

NCLEX item type: multiple response
Cognitive skill: application

29. The nurse reviewed what types of medications that can be applied to mucous membranes and recognized that they are available in which dose forms? *(Select all that apply.)* *(83)*
    1. Sublingual tablets
    2. Suppository
    3. Transdermal disk
    4. Dry powder inhaler
    5. Buccal tablets

Objective: Compare the techniques used to administer eardrops to patients who are less than 3 years old with that used for patients who are 3 years and older.

NCLEX item type: multiple choice
Cognitive skill: interpret

30. When administering eardrops to a child younger than 3 years, the nurse should restrain the child, turn the head to the appropriate side, and gently pull the earlobe in which direction? *(92)*
    1. Downward and back
    2. Downward and forward
    3. Upward and back
    4. Upward and forward

NCLEX item type: multiple choice
Cognitive skill: comprehension

31. When applying eardrops to a child, the nurse notices that there is a large amount of wax buildup in the ear canal. What will the nurse do next? *(92)*
    1. Administer the medication, as the wax will not be a problem.
    2. Remove the wax with a cotton-tipped applicator prior to administration.
    3. Obtain an order to gently remove wax by irrigating the ear canal prior to administration.
    4. Call the healthcare provider and ask for another route for the medication to be administered.

Objective: Describe the purpose, the precautions necessary, and the patient education required for those patients who require medications via inhalation.

NCLEX item type: multiple response
Cognitive skill: compare

32. Which types of medications are available in the oral inhalation dose form? *(Select all that apply.)* *(96)*
    1. Bronchodilators
    2. Fentanyl
    3. Nitroglycerin
    4. Corticosteroids
    5. Allergens

NCLEX item type: multiple response
Cognitive skill: application

33. What does the nurse instruct the patient to do when administering medications via the inhalation route? *(Select all that apply.)* *(97)*
    1. Inhale deeply over 10 seconds after activating the MDI.
    2. Shake the medication canister before using MDIs.
    3. Rinse their mouth before using an inhaled corticosteroid.
    4. Blow into the dry powder inhaler (DPI).
    5. Place one end of the extender in the mouth and close the lips around it.

Objective: Identify the equipment needed, the site, and the specific techniques required to administer vaginal medications or douches.

NCLEX item type: multiple response
Cognitive skill: ordering

34. List in order the steps the nurse takes to administer a vaginal suppository. *(98-99)*
    1. _____ Perform hand hygiene and don gloves.
    2. _____ Lubricate the gloved index finger and insert the suppository.
    3. _____ Ask the patient to void prior to administration.
    4. _____ Place the patient in the correct position and unwrap a vaginal suppository that has been warmed to room temperature, and lubricate it with a water-soluble lubricant.
    5. _____ Document the administration.

Copyright © 2023 by Elsevier, Inc. All rights reserved.

NCLEX item type: multiple choice
Cognitive skill: explain

35. In what position should the nurse place a patient who is to be administered a vaginal medication? *(98)*
    1. On the left side
    2. On the back with legs in the air
    3. On the stomach with knees tucked
    4. On the back in the lithotomy position

NCLEX item type: multiple choice
Cognitive skill: comprehension

36. The nurse instructed the patient on when douching is recommended for which use? *(98)*
    1. When there is a vaginal infection present
    2. As a normal feminine hygiene practice
    3. As an effective method of birth control
    4. After a vaginal suppository has been administered

Copyright © 2023 by Elsevier, Inc. All rights reserved.

Enteral Administration

Answer Key: Textbook page references are provided as a guide for answering these questions. A complete answer key is provided to your instructor.

MATCHING

Match the term on the right with the definition on the left.

Definition

1. _____ medication dissolved in a concentrated solution of sugar and water
2. _____ medication dissolved in alcohol and water
3. _____ small, cylindrical gelatin containers that hold dry powder or liquid medication
4. _____ dry powdered medication compressed into small disks
5. _____ liquids with solid insoluble drug particles dispersed solution, requires shaking prior to use
6. _____ flat disks in a sugar base form to dissolve slowly in the mouth
7. _____ dispersion of small droplets of water in oil by means of an emulsifying agent

Term

a. tablet
b. capsule
c. lozenge
d. elixir
e. emulsion
f. syrup
g. suspension

REVIEW QUESTIONS

Objective: Describe general principles of administering solid forms of oral medications.
NCLEX item type: multiple response
Cognitive skill: application

8. The nurse reviewed the *enteral route* of administration which involves giving medications directly into the gastrointestinal (GI) tract; this includes which example? *(Select all that apply.)* **(103)**
   1. Rectally
   2. Orally
   3. Sublingually
   4. Gastrointestinal (GI) tube
   5. Percutaneous endoscopic gastrostomy (PEG) or G tube

NCLEX item type: multiple response
Cognitive skill: explain

9. The nurse identified the advantages of the oral route of medication administration with a patient and included which statement? *(Select all that apply.)* **(103)**
   1. "It is easy to administer medications orally."
   2. "This route has a slow absorption rate."
   3. "This route is the most economical."
   4. "The oral route is the most convenient."
   5. "It is easy to retrieve medications orally, if given in error."

NCLEX item type: multiple response
Cognitive skill: application

10. When administering a solid form of medication to a patient, which procedures does the nurse apply? *(Select all that apply.)* **(108)**
    1. Using a tablet-crushing device for appropriate medications when patients have difficulty swallowing
    2. Having the patient place the medication on the front of the tongue
    3. Encouraging the patient to keep the head back while swallowing
    4. Remaining with the patient while the medication is being taken
    5. Having the patient drink a full glass of water with the medication

Objective: Compare the different techniques that are used with a unit-dose distribution system and an electronic controlled distribution system.
NCLEX item type: multiple choice
Cognitive skill: compare

11. Which system requires the nurse to use a security access code and password? **(107)**
    1. Electronic controlled system
    2. Medication card system
    3. Unit-dose distribution system
    4. Medication administration record system

Copyright © 2023 by Elsevier, Inc. All rights reserved.

NCLEX item type: multiple choice
Cognitive skill: relate

12. When distributing medications via the computer-controlled system, what will the nurse need to verify the medication? *(107)*
    1. The medication profile
    2. A medication card
    3. Another nurse to verify the correct dosage
    4. The patient to correctly identify the medication

NCLEX item type: multiple choice
Cognitive skill: understand

13. Which system is designed to allow the nurse to hand the medication to the patient and allow him or her to read the package label? *(107)*
    1. Computer-controlled system
    2. Unit-dose system
    3. Medication administration record
    4. Medication card system

Objective: Identify general principles used for liquid-form oral medication administration.

NCLEX item type: multiple choice
Cognitive skill: contrast

14. To read the correct amount of a liquid medication that has been poured into a medicine cup, the nurse reads the meniscus at which point? *(109)*
    1. At the lowest point of the convex curve in the cup
    2. At the highest point of the concave curve in the cup
    3. At the lowest point of the concave curve in the cup
    4. At the highest point of the convex curve in the cup

NCLEX item type: multiple choice
Cognitive skill: compare

15. The nurse remembers that the term for small droplets of water in oil or oil in water that are used to mask bitter tastes or provide better solubility to certain drugs is knows as what? *(105)*
    1. An elixir
    2. A suspension
    3. A syrup
    4. An emulsion

NCLEX item type: multiple choice
Cognitive skill: comprehension

16. When administering a liquid form of an oral medication to an infant, what does the nurse need to confirm? *(110)*
    1. That the infant is alert
    2. That the infant is positioned so that the head is lowered
    3. That the syringe or dropper is at the tip of the infant's tongue
    4. That the medicine is given rapidly to facilitate swallowing of the medicine

Objective: Cite the equipment needed, techniques used, and precautions necessary when administering medications via gastrointestinal tubes.

NCLEX item type: multiple response
Cognitive skill: application

17. The alternative route of giving medications by GI tube is generally done because the patient has which condition? *(Select all that apply.)* *(110)*
    1. The patient is comatose.
    2. The patient is unable to swallow.
    3. The patient has had back surgery.
    4. The patient has a disorder of the esophagus.
    5. The patient refuses to take medications orally.

NCLEX item type: multiple response
Cognitive skill: ordering

18. List in order the proper procedure the nurse will use for administration of a drug via a GI tube. *(112)*
    1. _____ Clamp the tubing at the end of medication administration.
    2. _____ Position the patient upright and check the location of the GI tube.
    3. _____ Flush the tube with 30 mL of water using a larger syringe.
    4. _____ Perform hand hygiene and don gloves.
    5. _____ Document the medication and how the patient tolerated the procedure.

NCLEX item type: multiple response
Cognitive skill: application

19. Why should the nurse flush the GI tube after administration of enteral formulas? *(Select all that apply.)* *(113)*
    1. To remove the formula from the tubing
    2. To maintain the patency of the tube
    3. To allow better absorption of the formula from the stomach
    4. To ensure the tube stays in position after the feeding
    5. To prevent the formula remaining in the tube from supporting bacterial growth

NCLEX item type: multiple choice
Cognitive skill: comprehension

20. When working with patients receiving intermittent enteral feedings via a gastrostomy tube, which position does the patient need to be in? *(113)*
    1. The lithotomy position
    2. The semi-Fowler's position
    3. The prone position
    4. The supine position

Copyright © 2023 by Elsevier, Inc. All rights reserved.

Objective: Cite the equipment needed and the technique required when administering rectal suppositories and disposable enemas.

NCLEX item type: multiple choice

Cognitive skill: explain

21. What instructions will the nurse give the patient when administering a rectal suppository? *(114)*
    1. "Hold your breath while I insert the suppository."
    2. "Get out of bed as soon as I get the suppository in place."
    3. "Try to hold the suppository for 15-20 minutes."
    4. "You will need to lay on your right side before I can insert this suppository."

NCLEX item type: multiple choice

Cognitive skill: evaluate

22. How should the nurse administer rectal suppository medications? *(114)*
    1. They should be self-administered.
    2. Ask another nurse to give, as it is not pleasant to do.
    3. Discard the medication if a suppository becomes soft.
    4. Administer when the patient is lying on the left side.

NCLEX item type: multiple response

Cognitive skill: ordering

23. List in order the procedure for administration that the nurse uses for a disposable enema. *(115)*
    1. _____ Check pertinent patient monitoring parameters (i.e., last time defecated).
    2. _____ Explain carefully to the patient the procedure for administering an enema.
    3. _____ Put on gloves, remove protective covering from the rectal tube, and lubricate.
    4. _____ Position the patient on the left side and drape.
    5. _____ Remove and discard gloves and wash hands thoroughly.

NCLEX item type: multiple choice

Cognitive skill: comprehension

24. When administering an enema to an adult, what does the nurse do? *(115)*
    1. Encourages the patient to hold the solution for about 5 minutes before defecating
    2. Heats the enema to 101° F to ensure comfort in administration
    3. Inserts 1 inch of the lubricated rectal tube into the rectum
    4. Tells the patient not to flush the toilet until the nurse returns and can see the results of the enema

Copyright © 2023 by Elsevier, Inc. All rights reserved.

Parenteral Administration: Safe Preparation of Parenteral Medications

chapter

9

Answer Key: Textbook page references are provided as a guide for answering these questions. A complete answer key is provided to your instructor.

MATCHING

Match the key term on the left with the definition on the right

Key Term

1. _____ prefilled cartridges and syringes
2. _____ needle gauge
3. _____ safety devices
4. _____ plunger
5. _____ Mix-O-Vials
6. _____ milliliter scale
7. _____ ampules

Definition

a. glass containers usually contain a single dose of a medication
b. represents the units whereby medications are routinely ordered
c. medication supplied in a premeasured amount
d. the diameter of the hole through the needle
e. products developed for syringes and needles to prevent sharps injuries
f. glass containers with two components
g. the inner cylindrical portion the fits snugly in the barrel

REVIEW QUESTIONS

Objective: Identify safe administration practices for parenteral medications.

NCLEX item type: multiple choice
Cognitive skill: comprehension

8. The nurse is preparing to give a subcutaneous injection of 0.5 mL of dalteparin. The medication should be injected using which syringe? *(122)*
   1. An insulin syringe
   2. A tuberculin syringe
   3. A prefilled syringe
   4. A standard plastic syringe

NCLEX item type: multiple choice
Cognitive skill: knowledge

9. The nurse knows that insulin syringes are specifically calibrated to measure what? *(121)*
   1. Doses of epinephrine
   2. Any volume smaller than 1 mL
   3. Volumes for tuberculin inoculations
   4. Doses of insulin only

NCLEX item type: multiple response
Cognitive skill: application

10. What does the nurse instructing the patient on the use of an insulin pen include in the teaching? *(Select all that apply.) (122)*
    1. How to hold the pen correctly
    2. How to dial in the correct amount of insulin
    3. When to replace the cartridge
    4. How to measure the dose with a tuberculin syringe
    5. Which site to insert the needle

NCLEX item type: multiple choice
Cognitive skill: knowledge

11. The nurse explains the use of the low-dose insulin syringes to a patient, and stated that they are used to measure insulin up to what dose? *(121)*
    1. 100 units
    2. 50 units
    3. 25 unit
    4. 10 units

NCLEX item type: multiple choice
Cognitive skill: comprehension

12. The nurse recognizes that the difference between a safety syringe and an ordinary syringe is that the safety syringe has which attachment? *(126)*
    1. The sleeve or sheath
    2. The needle cover
    3. The calibration measure
    4. The plunger topper

Copyright © 2023 by Elsevier, Inc. All rights reserved.

NCLEX item type: multiple choice
Cognitive skill: analysis

13. Two nurses were in the medication room discussing the difference between the volume of medication that can be given in any subcutaneous site and the intradermal site. Which statement is correct? *(124)*
    1. "I always give between 0.5 mL and 1 mL for intradermal, and less than 0.1 mL for subcutaneous injections."
    2. "I always give between 0.01 mL and 0.1 mL for intradermal, and less than 1 mL for subcutaneous injections."
    3. "I always give between 0.01 mL and 0.1 mL for intradermal, and less than 2 mL for subcutaneous injections."
    4. "I always give between 0.1 mL and 1 mL for intradermal, and less than 0.5 mL for subcutaneous injections."

Objective: Compare and contrast the volumes of medications that can be measured in a tuberculin syringe and those of larger-volume syringes.

NCLEX item type: multiple choice
Cognitive skill: interpret

14. The nurse is preparing to administer an intramuscular (IM) injection of 1 mg of Haldol, which comes in a concentration of 1 mg/1 mL, to a confused patient. In the medication room, the nurse is choosing the correct needle and syringe from the shelf. The patient was an adult of normal weight, so the nurse selected which syringe? *(120)*
    1. a 5-mL syringe
    2. a 3-mL syringe
    3. a 10-mL syringe
    4. a tuberculin syringe

NCLEX item type: multiple choice
Cognitive skill: relate

15. The nurse understands that the use of the tuberculin syringe is limited because it can only be used for what? *(120)*
    1. Tuberculin inoculations
    2. Volumes smaller than 1 mL
    3. Insulin administration
    4. Volumes greater than 1 mL

NCLEX-NG item type: matrix/grid
Cognitive skill: take action

16. The nurse in the medication room was preparing to administer multiple injections to several patients. Which syringe does the nurse chose for each order? *(120-121)*

Indicate with an 'X' in the box which syringe would be appropriate for each type of injection ordered.

	3 mL syringe	Tuberculin syringe	Regular dose insulin	Low dose insulin
Insulin dose of 55 units				
IM injection of 0.5 mL				
Insulin dose of 20 units				
Subcutaneous injection of 1 mL				
Intradermal injection of 0.05 mL				

Objective: Describe how to select the correct needle gauge and length.

NCLEX item type: multiple choice
Cognitive skill: knowledge

17. The nurse knows that the gauge of the needle is marked on the hub of the needle and on the outside of the disposable package; what does this number represent? *(124)*
    1. The length of the needle
    2. The inner diameter of the needle
    3. The actual dose the needle can hold
    4. The maximum volume allowed when using this needle

NCLEX item type: multiple choice
Cognitive skill: comprehension

18. When preparing to administer an intradermal injection the nurse will select which gauge and length of needle? *(124)*
    1. 25 gauge; 5/8 inch
    2. 18 gauge; 1 inch
    3. 29 gauge; 3/8 inch
    4. 20 gauge; 1/2 inch

Copyright © 2023 by Elsevier, Inc. All rights reserved.

NCLEX item type: multiple choice
Cognitive skill: classify

19. What factor does the nurse base the selection of the proper needle gauge on? *(124)*
    1. The dose of the medication
    2. The site of injection
    3. The viscosity (thickness) of the solution
    4. The calibration scale used

Objective: Compare and contrast the advantages and disadvantages of using prefilled syringes.
NCLEX item type: multiple response
Cognitive skill: contrast

20. The nurse knows that the *advantages* of using a prefilled syringe include which factors? *(Select all that apply.) (122)*
    1. These syringes are to be used once and discarded.
    2. The time that is saved in preparing a standard amount of medication for one injection.
    3. The nurse can expect these syringes are cheaper than multi-dose vials.
    4. There is decreased chance for contamination using these syringes.
    5. A cartridge is required for use to hold the prefilled syringe.

NCLEX item type: multiple response
Cognitive skill: compare

21. The nurse knows that the *disadvantages* of using a prefilled syringe include which factors? *(Select all that apply.) (122)*
    1. The nurse does not draw up the medication.
    2. An additional medication generally cannot be added to the cartridge.
    3. These syringes are to be used once and discarded.
    4. A cartridge is required for use to hold the prefilled syringe.
    5. The nurse can expect that these syringes are more expensive than multi-vials.

NCLEX item type: multiple response
Cognitive skill: application

22. Many hospital pharmacies will use prefilled syringes for specific doses of medication for some patients, including what examples? *(Select all that apply.) (122)*
    1. Carpuject syringes
    2. Insulin pens
    3. Plastic syringes
    4. Tuberculin syringes
    5. EpiPen

Objective: Differentiate among ampules, vials, and Mix-O-Vials.
NCLEX item type: multiple choice
Cognitive skill: illustrate

23. The nurse explains to a nursing student that the glass containers that may be scored or have a darkened ring around the neck and usually contain a single dose of a medication are called what? *(126)*
    1. Ampules
    2. Metal lid vial
    3. Mix-O-Vials
    4. Rubber diaphragm vials

NCLEX item type: multiple choice
Cognitive skill: explain

24. The nurse explains to the nursing student that the glass or plastic containers that contain one or more doses of a sterile medication are called what? *(126-127)*
    1. Vials
    2. Scored ampules
    3. Mix-O-Vials
    4. Ringed ampules

NCLEX item type: multiple choice
Cognitive skill: interpret

25. How does the nurse use a Mix-O-Vial? (A single dose of medication is normally contained in the Mix-O-Vial.) *(128)*
    1. By applying pressure to the rubber stopper between the two chambers
    2. By applying pressure to the top rubber diaphragm plunger
    3. By shaking the upper chamber (which contains the solvent) until it falls into the lower chamber (which contains the drug)
    4. By shaking the lower chamber (which contains the drug) until the upper chamber (which contains the solvent) falls down into the lower chamber

Objective: Describe the technique used to prepare two different drugs in one syringe (e.g., insulin).
NCLEX item type: multiple choice
Cognitive skill: comprehension

26. When preparing NPH and Regular insulin together in the same syringe, what does the nurse need to do? *(132)*
    1. Discards NPH insulin if it is cloudy
    2. First draws up the NPH insulin to be administered
    3. First inject the amount of air equal to the amount of insulin to be withdrawn into the Regular insulin
    4. Inject the first type of insulin already in the syringe into the second vial

Copyright © 2023 by Elsevier, Inc. All rights reserved.

NCLEX item type: multiple response
Cognitive skill: application

27. The nurse is preparing to administer 58 units of insulin and knows that which is true regarding insulin syringes? *(Select all that apply.)* **(121)**
    1. The shorter lines on the Regular insulin syringe represent 2 units measured.
    2. The longer lines on the low-dose insulin syringe measure 10 units of insulin.
    3. The low-dose insulin syringe can be used for this dose.
    4. The longer lines on the Regular insulin syringe measure 5 units of insulin.
    5. The shorter lines on the low-dose insulin syringe represent 1 unit measured.

NCLEX item type: multiple response
Cognitive skill: ordering

28. List in order the correct sequence the nurse will follow to mix NPH and Regular insulin. **(132)**
    1. _____ Insert the needle into the NPH vial, and withdraw the correct amount of insulin.
    2. _____ Inject air into the Regular vial, invert the bottle, and withdraw the correct amount of Regular insulin.
    3. _____ Fill the syringe with air to an amount equal to the correct amount of NPH, insert the needle into the vial, inject air, remove needle without withdrawing any insulin.
    4. _____ Check the insulin prescription and wipe the tops of both vials of insulin.
    5. _____ Fill the syringe with air to an amount equal to the correct amount of Regular insulin.

Copyright © 2023 by Elsevier, Inc. All rights reserved.

Parenteral Administration: Intradermal, Subcutaneous, and Intramuscular Routes

Answer Key: Textbook page references are provided as a guide for answering these questions. A complete answer key is provided to your instructor.

MATCHING
Match the description on the right with the intramuscular site on the left.

Intramuscular Site

1. _____ vastus lateralis

2. _____ ventrogluteal

3. _____ rectus femoris

4. _____ deltoid

Description

a. Considered easiest site when patients are sitting

b. Considered easiest site for self-administration

c. Considered the preferred IM site for infants

d. Considered easiest site when patients are side-lying

REVIEW QUESTIONS

Objective: Describe the technique that is used to administer a medication via the intradermal route.
NCLEX item type: multiple choice
Cognitive skill: comprehension

5. The nurse explains to the patient the most common site for the administration of intradermal medication is the inner aspect of which body part? *(137)*
   1. The shin
   2. The thigh
   3. The forearm
   4. The upper arm

NCLEX item type: multiple response
Cognitive skill: application

6. When administering intradermal allergy testing for a patient, which steps does the nurse perform? *(Select all that apply.) (138-139)*
   1. Uses an alcohol wipe to clean the skin
   2. Wipes the site with alcohol after injection
   3. Aspirates for blood once the needle has been inserted
   4. Injects the volume ordered, usually 0.01-0.05 mL, into the subcutaneous tissue
   5. Asks the patient if any antihistamine or anti-inflammatory agents were taken 24-48 hours before the test

NCLEX item type: multiple choice
Cognitive skill: interpret

7. When preparing to provide allergy testing to a patient using the intradermal injection technique, what does the nurse do? *(138)*
   1. Performs hand hygiene and applies gloves
   2. Inserts the needle at a 90-degree angle with the needle bevel facing down
   3. Recaps the used needle before disposing of it in a puncture-resistant container
   4. Deposits the solution being injected into the subcutaneous tissue

Objective: Identify the equipment needed, and describe the technique that is used to administer a medication via the subcutaneous route.
NCLEX item type: multiple choice
Cognitive skill: analyze

8. The nurse is teaching a patient about the importance of rotating subcutaneous insulin injection sites. Which statement made by the patient indicates a need for additional teaching? *(140)*
   1. "The fastest site of absorption is when I inject into the abdomen."
   2. "Exercise will not affect the rate of insulin absorption."
   3. "Common subcutaneous sites for administering insulin include upper arms, anterior thighs, and the abdomen."
   4. "I need to rotate injection sites to prevent lipohypertrophy, which will slow insulin absorption."

Copyright © 2023 by Elsevier, Inc. All rights reserved.

NCLEX item type: multiple choice
Cognitive skill: knowledge
9. The nurse knows which route of injection is considered the fastest for medication absorption? *(141)*
   1. Intradermal
   2. Intraocular
   3. Subcutaneous
   4. Intramuscular

NCLEX item type: multiple choice
Cognitive skill: interpret
10. The nurse was educating a patient about heparin injections that would need to be continued at home, and the patient states, "I know that I need to inject my abdominal area just under the skin, right?" How should the nurse respond? *(140)*
    1. "That's correct, this is an intradermal injection."
    2. "Actually, this injection will go into the subcutaneous tissue, or the fat that is under the skin."
    3. "Well, this injection is designed to be delivered into your muscle, so instead of the abdomen, you will give it in your leg."
    4. "That is almost correct. It will go under your skin, but not in your abdomen; it will be in your arm."

Objective: Describe the techniques used to administer medications intramuscularly.
NCLEX item type: multiple choice
Cognitive skill: comprehension
11. The nurse is preparing to administer an IM injection in the ventrogluteal area. What does the nurse do first? *(142-143)*
    1. Positions the patient supine with the toes pointed inward
    2. Have the patient flex the gluteal muscle to minimize pain from the injection
    3. Identifies the site by forming a "V" on the lateral portion of the greater trochanter
    4. The needle needs to be inserted at a 30-degree angle to the surface of the patient's skin

NCLEX item type: multiple response
Cognitive skill: ordering
12. List the steps in order that the nurse will follow to administer an IM injection. *(144)*
    1. _____ Apply a small bandage to the site.
    2. _____ Explain carefully to the patient what will be done.
    3. _____ Insert the needle at the correct angle and depth for the site being used.
    4. _____ Carefully identify the patient using two patient identifiers.
    5. _____ Provide for privacy; position the patient appropriately.

NCLEX item type: multiple choice
Cognitive skill: comprehension
13. What is the most important instruction to follow for the nurse administering an IM injection? *(143)*
    1. Add a bubble of air to the syringe.
    2. Pinch the skin into a bunch prior to injection.
    3. Tell the patient to hold his breath during the injection.
    4. Correctly identify the patient prior to administration.

Objective: Describe the landmarks that are used to identify the vastus lateralis muscle, the rectus femoris muscle, the ventrogluteal area, and the deltoid muscle before medication is administered.
NCLEX item type: multiple choice
Cognitive skill: knowledge
14. When administering an IM injection in the deltoid muscle, the nurse will locate the site using which landmarks? *(143)*
    1. Finding the anterior lateral thigh
    2. Placing one hands-breadth below the greater trochanter
    3. Palpating the top of the shoulder and measuring down three finger-breadths
    4. From the crest of the ilium, directing the needle slightly upward

NCLEX item type: multiple choice
Cognitive skill: compare
15. Which site for injection is located by placing the palm of the hand on the lateral portion of the greater trochanter, the thumb pointing toward the groin, the index finger on the anterior superior iliac spine, and the middle finger extended to the iliac crest? *(143)*
    1. The rectus femoris muscle
    2. The deltoid muscle
    3. The vastus lateralis muscle
    4. The ventrogluteal muscle

NCLEX item type: multiple choice
Cognitive skill: understand
16. The nurse recognizes that the location of the vastus lateralis muscle is where? *(142)*
    1. In the buttock area
    2. On the thigh
    3. Below the shoulder
    4. Under the armpit

Copyright © 2023 by Elsevier, Inc. All rights reserved.

Objective: Identify suitable sites for the intramuscular administration of medication in an infant, a child, an adult, and an older adult.

NCLEX item type: multiple choice

Cognitive skill: explain

17. The nurse educated the mother of an infant where the best site for an IM injection was for her infant and mentioned which muscle? *(142)*
    1. The deltoid
    2. The rectus femoris
    3. The vastus lateralis
    4. The ventrogluteal

NCLEX item type: multiple choice

Cognitive skill: comprehension

18. The nurse is planning to administer an IM injection for an adult patient who needs a flu vaccine (0.5 mL). Which muscle is the best to use? *(143)*
    1. The deltoid muscle
    2. The rectus femoris muscle
    3. The vastus lateralis muscle
    4. The ventrogluteal muscle

NCLEX item type: multiple response

Cognitive skill: application

19. What does the nurse need to do before administering an IM injection into an older adult? *(Select all that apply.) (143-144)*
    1. Check the patient's allergy list.
    2. Verify the patient's identity using two identifiers.
    3. Cleanse the skin with an alcohol wipe.
    4. Ask another nurse to verify the correct dose prior to administration.
    5. Insert the needle to a depth of 1/2 inch and inject the medication.

Copyright © 2023 by Elsevier, Inc. All rights reserved.

Parenteral Administration: Intravenous Route

chapter **11**

Answer Key: Textbook page references are provided as a guide for answering these questions. A complete answer key is provided to your instructor.

MATCHING

Match the definition on the right with the complication on the left.

Complication

1. _____ extravasation
2. _____ infiltration
3. _____ speed shock
4. _____ thrombophlebitis
5. _____ pulmonary edema
6. _____ septicemia
7. _____ localized infection
8. _____ phlebitis

Definition

a. symptoms include dyspnea, cough, coarse crackles, and frothy sputum
b. pathogens from a local infection invade the bloodstream causing fever and chills
c. an inflammation of a vein
d. the leakage of an intravenous solution into the surrounding tissue
e. redness, warmth, purulent drainage, swelling, and burning pain along the course of the vein
f. the leakage of an irritating chemical into the surrounding tissue
g. an inflammation of a vein with an associated blood clot
h. flushing, tightness in the chest, and hypotension

REVIEW QUESTIONS

Objective: Discuss the different IV access devices used for IV therapy.

NCLEX item type: multiple choice
Cognitive skill: knowledge

9. The nurse explains to the patient with an implanted port that there are different types of needles that are used to access the port, and described which kind? *(155)*
   1. Huber needles
   2. Subclavian needles
   3. Hickman needles
   4. Intravenous needles

NCLEX item type: multiple response
Cognitive skill: illustrate

10. What supplies does the nurse preparing to start an IV on a patient need? *(Select all that apply.) (163)*
    1. Sterile gloves
    2. Alcohol wipes
    3. Tourniquet
    4. Transparent dressing
    5. IV catheter

NCLEX item type: multiple response
Cognitive skill: application

11. The nurse knows that the common locations for peripheral IVs include which veins? *(Select all that apply.) (158)*
    1. The metacarpal veins
    2. The dorsal veins
    3. The jugular veins
    4. The basilic veins
    5. The cephalic veins

NCLEX item type: multiple response
Cognitive skill: application

12. When a patient needs long-term IV or home IV therapy, the nurse knows that the various types of catheters used will include which types? *(Select all that apply.) (154)*
    1. Peripherally inserted central catheters (PICC)
    2. Tunneled central venous catheters
    3. Implantable venous access devices
    4. Peripheral saline locks
    5. Hickman or Broviac catheters

Copyright © 2023 by Elsevier, Inc. All rights reserved.

NCLEX item type: multiple choice
Cognitive skill: contrast

13. The nurse explained to the patient where PICC lines can be inserted and made which correct statement? *(154)*
    1. "PICC lines are inserted in the jugular vein and threaded down to end at the superior vena cava."
    2. "PICC lines are inserted in the cephalic vein and threaded down to end at the superior vena cava."
    3. "PICC lines are inserted in the subclavian vein and threaded down to end at the superior vena cava."
    4. "PICC lines are inserted in the metacarpal vein and threaded down to end at the superior vena cava."

Objective: Differentiate among isotonic, hypotonic, and hypertonic IV solutions and explain their clinical uses.

NCLEX item type: multiple choice
Cognitive skill: comprehension

14. A patient has been admitted to the healthcare facility after experiencing a GI bleed at home, which has now resolved. The patient now has an intravascular fluid volume deficit. Which IV fluid does the nurse anticipate will be prescribed for the patient? *(156)*
    1. 0.9% sodium chloride
    2. 0.2% sodium chloride
    3. 0.45% sodium chloride
    4. 5% dextrose in 0.2% sodium chloride

NCLEX item type: multiple choice
Cognitive skill: illustrate

15. The nurse recognizes that hypertonic solutions (e.g., parenteral nutrition solutions) are administered through central infusion lines directly into which blood vessel? *(157)*
    1. The cephalic veins
    2. The basilic veins
    3. The temporal veins
    4. The superior vena cava

NCLEX item type: multiple choice
Cognitive skill: understanding

16. The nurse remembers learning about IV solutions and those that contain fewer electrolytes and more free water are known as what? *(156)*
    1. Isotonic
    2. Hypotonic
    3. Hypertonic
    4. Replacement solutions

Objective: Identify the general principles for administering medications via the IV route.

NCLEX item type: multiple response
Cognitive skill: compare

17. The nurse prepared to administer IV medications which are available in what dose forms? *(Select all that apply.)* *(157)*
    1. Vials
    2. Tablets
    3. Prefilled syringes
    4. Ampules
    5. Large-volume IV solution bags

NCLEX item type: multiple response
Cognitive skill: application

18. In general, what does the nurse need to consider regarding any medication administered via the IV route? *(Select all that apply.)* *(160)*
    1. The SAS technique
    2. When an inline filter is needed
    3. Use of appropriate barrier precautions
    4. Topical antibiotic creams are to be used on all insertion sites
    5. Used needles, syringes, and access devices are placed in puncture-resistant containers

NCLEX item type: multiple response
Cognitive skill: interpret

19. The nurse knows there are various IV catheters used for IV administration and include which types? *(Select all that apply.)* *(153,154)*
    1. PICCs
    2. Midline catheters
    3. Peripheral venous catheters
    4. Central venous catheters
    5. Arterial catheters

Objective: Compare and contrast the differences between a peripheral IV line and a central IV line.

NCLEX item type: multiple response
Cognitive skill: application

20. The nurse is reviewing the different types of peripheral IV devices with an orientee and indicated which ones are examples of peripheral IV access devices? *(Select all that apply.)* *(153)*
    1. Midline access catheters
    2. Saline lock
    3. PICCs
    4. Infusion ports
    5. Tunneled catheters

Copyright © 2023 by Elsevier, Inc. All rights reserved.

NCLEX item type: multiple choice
Cognitive skill: explain

21. The nurse was teaching a patient about the need for a central IV access device and recognized further teaching was needed when the patient made which statement? *(154)*
    1. "I guess my veins in my arms are shot from the repeated IVs I have had, so a central line makes sense."
    2. "Since I will need to have long-term antibiotic therapy, it makes sense to have a PICC line."
    3. "I understand about Port-a-Caths since my wife's cousin had one for her chemotherapy."
    4. "As I understand it, this will mean that I will need to have my PICC changed every 3 months."

NCLEX item type: multiple response
Cognitive skill: compare

22. The nurse compares the advantages of a peripheral IV with an central IV when teaching the patient. Which statements by the nurse need to be revised? *(Select all that apply.) (154)*
    1. "The peripheral IV line has fewer complications than the central IV line."
    2. "The peripheral IV line is easier to insert than the central IV line."
    3. "The peripheral IV line lasts longer than the central IV line."
    4. "The peripheral IV line costs less than the central IV line."
    5. "The peripheral IV line requires saline flushes while most central IV lines require heparin."

NCLEX item type: multiple choice
Cognitive skill: comprehension

23. A patient has been ordered a PICC for the administration of medications. The nurse has taught the patient about the insertion procedure, use, and care of the PICC line. Which statement made by the patient indicates a need for further teaching? *(153-154)*
    1. "I will be able to go home with a PICC line."
    2. "My PICC line can last up to a year if it is properly cared for."
    3. "I will be placed under general anesthesia to have this intravenous line inserted."
    4. "The PICC line should be flushed with a saline-heparin solution after every use, or daily if not used."

Objective: Describe the correct techniques for administering medications by means of a saline lock, an IV bag, an infusion pump, and a secondary piggyback set.

NCLEX item type: multiple response
Cognitive skill: ordering

24. The nurse follows which steps in order when administering a medication by a saline lock? *(Select all that apply.) (166-167)*
    1. Selects a syringe several milliliters larger than that required by the volume of the drug.
    2. After determining that the IV has a blood return, injects saline for the flush followed by the medication at the rate specified by the manufacturer.
    3. After the medication is administered, inserts another syringe containing normal saline to flush the remaining drug from the catheter.
    4. Maintains constant pressure on the plunger of the syringe used to flush the line after the medication has been administered while simultaneously withdrawing the needle from the injection port to prevent backflow of blood.
    5. Draws up the correct amount of the medication in the syringe, and bring flush syringes to the patient's room.

NCLEX item type: multiple choice
Cognitive skill: evaluate

25. The nurse is hanging a bag of normal saline for a patient who has been diagnosed with dehydration, and notices that the peripheral IV that was placed in the patient's hand has become dislodged. What should the nurse do next? *(173-174)*
    1. Advance the catheter into the vein.
    2. Resecure the catheter to the patient's hand.
    3. Remove the catheter and insert another one.
    4. Use the catheter, as it should migrate back into place.

NCLEX item type: multiple response
Cognitive skill: application

26. While inserting an IV into a patient, the nurse has applied a tourniquet to help locate a vein. What other techniques are used in conjunction with a tourniquet to dilate the vein? *(Select all that apply.) (163)*
    1. Apply a heating pad.
    2. Apply cool, moist towels.
    3. Massage the vein.
    4. Place the extremity in a dependent position.
    5. Have the patient open and close his or her hand repeatedly.

Copyright © 2023 by Elsevier, Inc. All rights reserved.

Objective: Identify baseline assessments for IV therapy and proper maintenance of patency of IV lines and implanted access devices.

NCLEX item type: multiple choice

Cognitive skill: analyze

27. What are important teaching points for the nurse to cover for patients and family members when discussing maintenance of central lines? *(165)*
    1. Patients need to be taught the signs and symptoms of infection.
    2. Patients need to be taught how to document the dressing change.
    3. Patients need to be taught how to reinsert the catheter when it accidently comes out.
    4. Patients need to be taught to carefully wrap any sharps in tissue paper and discard in the trash.

NCLEX item type: multiple response

Cognitive skill: take action

28. When providing care to a patient receiving IV therapy, which actions does the nurse perform? *(Select all that apply.)* *(173-174)*
    1. Wears gloves to inspect the IV site
    2. Applies topical antibiotic ointment to the insertion site
    3. If it appears that the IV access device is clotted, attempts to clear the catheter by flushing with fluid
    4. Checks the drip chamber; if it is less than half full, squeezes it to fill more completely
    5. Checks the temperature of the solution being infused because cold solutions can cause spasms in the vein

NCLEX item type: multiple response

Cognitive skill: evaluate

29. The nurse is teaching the patient about their implantable infusion port. Which statement by the nurse needs to be corrected? *(Select all that apply.)* **(155)**
    1. Blood products can be administered through an implantable infusion port.
    2. One port of a two-port system may be reserved for drawing blood samples.
    3. An implanted central venous access catheter may remain in place for over a year and only requires a saline-heparin solution flush after every access or once monthly.
    4. The CDC recommends that central venous catheters be routinely replaced to prevent catheter-related infection.
    5. The infusion port can accommodate up to 100 punctures before it needs to be changed.

Objective: Explain the signs, symptoms, and treatment of the complications associated with IV therapy (e.g., phlebitis, thrombophlebitis, localized infection, septicemia, infiltration, extravasation, air in tubing, pulmonary edema, pulmonary embolism, and "speed shock").

NCLEX item type: multiple response

Cognitive skill: application

30. The nurse will monitor the patient with an IV for phlebitis, including which signs and symptoms? *(Select all that apply.)* **(174)**
    1. Streak formation over vein
    2. Erythema at insertion site
    3. Pain at insertion site
    4. Blanched skin around the insertion site
    5. Leaking from insertion site

NCLEX item type: multiple choice

Cognitive skill: analysis

31. What is the nurse concerned about when patients show signs of extravasation from IV drug drips or medications given IV push? *(175)*
    1. That serious tissue damage may occur
    2. That the patient will start to develop shortness of breath and hypotension
    3. That the patient is now developing an infection
    4. That the patient will experience warmth, tenderness, swelling, and burning pain in the IV site

NCLEX item type: cloze

Cognitive skill: recognize cues/take action

32. The nurse noted the patient with an IV running at 200 mL/hr started having signs and symptoms of circulatory overload which include _____1_____, _____1_____, _____1_____, and _____1_____. When these symptoms develop the nurse will position the patient in high Fowlers, and _____2_____, _____2_____, and _____2_____. *(176)*

Choose the most likely options for the information missing from the statements by selecting from the list of options provided.

Options for 1	Options for 2
Cyanosis	Start oxygen on the patient
Dyspnea	Obtain blood cultures
Sweating	Speed up the IV solution
Edema	Call the healthcare provider immediately
Engorged neck veins	Explain to the patient that they are experiencing speed shock
Fever	Remove the IV since it has become dislodged
Reduced urine output	Obtain vital signs

Copyright © 2023 by Elsevier, Inc. All rights reserved.

Drugs That Affect the Autonomic Nervous System

chapter
12

Answer Key: Textbook page references are provided as a guide for answering these questions. A complete answer key is provided to your instructor.

MATCHING
Match the definition in the right column with the key terms in the left column.

Key Term

1. _____ neurotransmitters
2. _____ catecholamines
3. _____ cholinergic agents
4. _____ anticholinergic agents
5. _____ adrenergic blocking agents
6. _____ adrenergic fibers
7. _____ cholinergic fibers
8. _____ central nervous system
9. _____ peripheral nervous system

Definition

a. the neurotransmitters -norepinephrine, epinephrine, and dopamine
b. nerve endings that secrete norepinephrine
c. medications that block the effects produced by the adrenergic neurotransmitter-norepinephrine
d. includes afferent and efferent nerves
e. nerve endings that liberate acetylcholine
f. medications that cause effects in the body similar to those produced by acetylcholine
g. includes the brain and the spinal cord
h. medications that block or inhibit cholinergic activity
i. chemical substances that either stimulate or inhibit electrical impulses through the neuron

REVIEW QUESTIONS

Scenario: A 69-year-old male was admitted to the hospital with an exacerbation of his asthma. He has a history of hypertension, diabetes, and benign prostatic hyperplasia (BPH). The patient is taking albuterol for his asthma, and metoprolol for his hypertension. He is taking currently controlled his diabetes with metformin, and takes Urecholine for the BPH.

Objective: Identify the most common neurotransmitters known toeffect central nervous system function.
NCLEX item type: multiple response
Cognitive skill: application

10. The nurse recalls that neurotransmitters that are released into synapses at the end of neurons are able to cause which reactions? *(Select all that apply.)* **(181)**
    1. They can secrete an enzyme.
    2. They can release a second neurotransmitter.
    3. They can stimulate receptors on an end organ.
    4. They can inhibit electrical impulses through the neuron.
    5. They can respond by transmitting a nerve signal.

NCLEX item type: multiple choice
Cognitive skill: comprehension

11. The nurse educated the patient on what happens when neurotransmitters are released into synaptic junctions, and made which correct statement? **(180)**
    1. "When a neurotransmitter is released a receptor is activated on the next neuron in the chain."
    2. "When a neurotransmitter is released a decrease in response to nerve stimulation occurs."
    3. "When a neurotransmitter is released the neurotransmitter activates the fight-or-flight response."
    4. "When a neurotransmitter is released the symptoms of Parkinson's disease become apparent."

NCLEX item type: multiple response
Cognitive skill: application

12. The nurse reviewed the major types of receptors found in the adrenergic side of the autonomic nervous system and determined that they include which type? *(Select all that apply.)* **(181)**
    1. Alpha
    2. Beta
    3. Dopaminergic
    4. Gamma
    5. Delta

Copyright © 2023 by Elsevier, Inc. All rights reserved.

NCLEX item type: multiple response
Cognitive skill: application
13. After reviewing the end-organ receptors that are part of the nervous system, the nurse recognizes which of these organs are usually at the end of the nerve chain? *(Select all that apply.)* **(180)**
    1. The brain
    2. The spinal cord
    3. The adrenal glands
    4. The heart muscle
    5. The smooth muscles of the GI tract

NCLEX item type: multiple choice
Cognitive skill: comprehension
14. The nurse discussed with the patient in the scenario that the medication used for asthma stimulates the beta adrenergic receptors in the lungs which causes which response from the receptors? **(181)**
    1. The smooth muscles of the lungs relax (open airways)
    2. The smooth muscles of the lungs contract (closes airways)
    3. The smooth muscles of the lungs secrete more mucous
    4. The smooth muscles of the lungs secrete less mucous

NCLEX item type: multiple choice
Cognitive skill: comprehension
15. The nurse reviews the nervous system which controls blood pressure and body temperature and recognizes this as which system? **(181)**
    1. Motor nervous system
    2. Voluntary nervous system
    3. Autonomic nervous system
    4. Somatic nervous system

Objective: Explain the actions of anticholinergic and beta-adrenergic blocking agents.
NCLEX item type: multiple choice
Cognitive skill: understanding
16. The nurse explains to the patient what is meant by an anticholinergic agent. Which statement by the nurse needs to be corrected? **(188)**
    1. "The anticholinergic agents are those medications that inhibit the action of the neurotransmitter acetylcholine."
    2. "Anticholinergic agents are used to stimulate cholinergic fibers."
    3. "Acetylcholine is a major neurotransmitter that is part of the autonomic nervous system."
    4. "When acetylcholine is released by the cholinergic fibers it causes the heart rate to slow. When you receive an anticholinergic it inhibits this effect."

NCLEX item type: multiple choice
Cognitive skill: understanding
17. The nurse explains to the patient what is meant by a beta-adrenergic blocking agent. Which statement by the nurse needs to be corrected? **(181,185)**
    1. "The part of the nervous system not under conscience or voluntary control called the adrenergic nervous system has alpha, beta, and dopamine receptors."
    2. "The beta-adrenergic blocking agents are those medications that block the beta receptors from being stimulated by neurotransmitters, such as norepinephrine and epinephrine."
    3. "When the beta receptors are blocked it causes the relaxation of the smooth muscles in the lungs."
    4. "The neurotransmitters that are involved with the adrenergic nervous system are norepinephrine, epinephrine, and dopamine."

NCLEX item type: grid
Cognitive skill: analyze cues
18. The nurse explains to a nursing student who was confused about the difference between anticholinergic and beta-blocking agents. Mark with an 'X' which class of agents have which effect. **(186, 188)**

Actions of the drugs	Anticholinergic agents	Beta-adrenergic blocking agents
Inhibits the relaxation of the smooth muscles in the lungs		
Inhibits cholinergic activity such as pupillary constriction		
Inhibits the adrenergic system		
Blocks the effects of acetylcholine		

Copyright © 2023 by Elsevier, Inc. All rights reserved.

Objective: Describe clinical uses and the predictable adverse effects of anticholinergic agents.

NCLEX item type: cloze
Cognitive skill: recognize cues

19. The nurse knows that anticholinergic agents are used clinically for _____1_____ and _____1_____ and have the predictable adverse effects of _____2_____ and _____2_____. *(188)*

Choose the most likely options for the information missing from the statements below by selecting from the list of options provided.

Opinion 1	Opinion 2
Reducing salivation	Increased blood pressure
Decreasing sweating	Blurred vision
Decrease heart rate	Dryness of the mucosa of the nose and mouth
Reducing urinary retention	Reduced hearing

NCLEX item type: multiple choice
Cognitive skill: interpret

20. The nurse explains to the patient the expected actions from anticholinergic agents. Which statement by the nurse needs to be corrected? *(188)*
    1. "Anticholinergic agents are medications that block the action of acetylcholine one of the major neurotransmitters in the nervous system."
    2. "The anticholinergic drugs have been associated with increased heart rate."
    3. "These drugs have the effect of inhibiting cholinergic activity result in decreasing secretions and decreasing the motility of the GI tract."
    4. "One of the effects of the anticholinergic drugs is that of pupil constriction."

NCLEX item type: multiple choice
Cognitive skill: understanding

21. The nurse is concerned about possible effects of administering anticholinergic agents to the patient in the scenario with a known enlarged prostate from BPH. Which of the following would be an example of an adverse effect? *(189)*
    1. Anticholinergics may cause an increase in urine production.
    2. Anticholinergics may cause an inability to void.
    3. Anticholinergics may cause episodes of incontinence.
    4. Anticholinergics may cause burning on urination.

Objective: Describe clinical uses and the predictable adverse effects of beta-adrenergic blocking agents.

NCLEX item type: multiple choice
Cognitive skill: understanding

22. The nurse knows that beta-adrenergic blocking agents such as carvedilol (Coreg) must be used with caution in diabetic patients because these agents may mask the signs of what? *(185)*
    1. Low urine output
    2. Tachycardia
    3. Hypoglycemia
    4. Hyperglycemia

NCLEX item type: multiple response
Cognitive skill: application

23. The patient in the scenario experiences orthostatic hypotension as a result of taking a beta-adrenergic blocking agent for treatment of hypertension. Which measures does the nurse incorporate into this patient's plan of care? *(Select all that apply.) (183,185)*
    1. Discontinue the beta-adrenergic-blocking agent.
    2. Instruct the patient to avoid standing for long periods.
    3. Encourage the patient to sit down if feeling faint.
    4. Teach the patient to rise slowly from a supine or sitting position.
    5. Teach the patient to perform exercises to prevent blood pooling in the extremities when standing or sitting for long periods.

NCLEX item type: multiple response
Cognitive skill: application

24. Since beta-adrenergic blocking agents have the potential to cause hypotension, bradycardia, and heart failure, it is important for the nurse to monitor for an increase in which symptoms of heart failure? *(Select all that apply.) (187)*
    1. Edema
    2. Crackles
    3. Dyspnea
    4. Urinary retention
    5. Hypoglycemia

NCLEX item type: multiple response
Cognitive skill: application

25. The nurse is aware of predictable adverse effects of beta-adrenergic blocking agent therapy and monitors the patient for which reaction? *(Select all that apply.) (187)*
    1. Nausea
    2. Bradycardia
    3. Wheezing
    4. Orthopnea
    5. Headache

Copyright © 2023 by Elsevier, Inc. All rights reserved.

Objective: Describe clinical uses and the predictable adverse effects of cholinergic agonists.

NCLEX item type: multiple choice
Cognitive skill: understanding

26. For patients who have benign prostatic hyperplasia and difficulty voiding, which class of drugs help by increasing contractions of the urinary bladder? *(188)*
    1. Anticholinergic agents
    2. Adrenergic agents
    3. Cholinergic agents
    4. Adrenergic-blocking agents

NCLEX item type: grid/matrix
Cognitive skill: evaluate cues

27. The nurse knows that since the cholinergic agents and the adrenergic agents have opposite effects. Indicate with an 'X' which effect is caused by which agents. *(188-189)*

	Cholinergic agents	Adrenergic agents
Pupillary constriction (miosis)		
Pupillary dilation (mydriasis)		
Slows heart rate		
Increased heart rate		
GI tract relaxes		

28. The nurse reviews the medications that the patient in the scenario was on: albuterol, metoprolol, and Urecholine. Which one is the cholinergic agent used clinically in the treatment of which disorder? *(188)*
    1. The albuterol for asthma
    2. The metoprolol for hypertension
    3. The Urecholine for urinary retention
    4. The metformin for diabetes

Objective: Describe clinical uses and the predictable adverse effects of adrenergic agonists.

NCLEX item type: multiple choice
Cognitive skill: understanding

29. During educating the patient in the scenario about their medications the patient made which statement that indicated to the nurse that further teaching is needed? *(182-183)*
    1. "I have been taking my albuterol for asthma now many years, and I have never had a problem with it."
    2. "I realize that the metoprolol I am taking may interfere with the effects of the albuterol but so far things are working fine."
    3. "I am not sure why there is any issue with my medications they have been working fine for me and I only get lightheaded and dizzy when I get up too fast from sitting."
    4. "I recognize that I did sometimes have palpitations and tremors with my meds but it went

away after awhile and I have not had any issues for quite some time now."

NCLEX item type: multiple choice
Cognitive skill: interpret

30. The patient mentioned to the nurse that they have recently started to feel nauseated and have vomiting on occasion without any apparent reason. The nurse responded appropriately by with which statement? *(183)*
    1. "I would not worry too much about it, I am sure it will pass."
    2. "I think we need to let your healthcare provider know about this recent development that may indicate your medications are causing you some trouble."
    3. "Have you taken anything for the nausea? I can recommend a few antiemetics."
    4. "Why do you think you are having this happen now? Are you having any family troubles?"

NCLEX-NG item type: cloze
Cognitive skill: recognize cues

31. The nurse knows that adrenergic agents are used clinically for _____1_____ and _____1_____ and have the predictable adverse effects of _____2_____ and _____2_____. *(181-183)*

Choose the most likely options for the information missing from the statements below by selecting from the list of options provided.

Option 1	Option 2
Emphysema	Urinary retention
Hypertension	Palpitations
Nasal congestion	Orthostatic hypotension
Dysrhythmias	Glaucoma

Copyright © 2023 by Elsevier, Inc. All rights reserved.

Drugs Used for Sedation and Sleep

Answer Key: Textbook page references are provided as a guide for answering these questions. A complete answer key is provided to your instructor.

MATCHING

Match the definition on the right with the sleep patterns on the left.

Sleep Pattern

1. _____ insomnia
2. _____ initial insomnia
3. _____ intermittent insomnia
4. _____ terminal insomnia
5. _____ short-term insomnia
6. _____ chronic insomnia
7. _____ rebound sleep

Definition

a. at least 1 month of sleep disturbance
b. the inability to fall asleep when desired
c. early awakening with the inability to fall asleep again
d. compensatory REM sleep
e. the inability to sleep
f. a sleep disturbance that lasts less than 3 weeks
g. the inability to stay asleep

REVIEW QUESTIONS

Scenario #1: A nurse taking care of a 58-year-old patient complaining of not being able to sleep, asked the patient if they were having trouble getting to sleep or if they woke up during the night and could not get back to sleep.

Objective: Differentiate among the terms *sedative* and *hypnotic; initial, intermittent,* and *terminal insomnia;* and *short-term* and *chronic insomnia* and *rebound sleep.*

NCLEX item type: multiple choice
Cognitive skill: compare

8. The nurse's questions to the patient in scenario #1 are intended to determine if there is which type of insomnia? *(193)*
   1. Initial insomnia or rebound insomnia
   2. Initial insomnia or intermittent insomnia
   3. Initial insomnia or terminal insomnia
   4. Initial insomnia or transient insomnia

NCLEX item type: multiple response
Cognitive skill: classify

9. The nurse knows which classification of drugs can be used for patients complaining of insomnia? *(Select all that apply.)* *(194)*
   1. Hypnotics
   2. Sedatives
   3. Antidepressants
   4. Anticonvulsants
   5. Anticholinergics

NCLEX item type: multiple choice
Cognitive skill: knowledge

10. The nurse knows that the phrase *rebound sleep* refers to what phenomenon? *(194)*
    1. The return to previous insomnia symptoms
    2. The increase in amount of REM sleep that causes restlessness and vivid nightmares
    3. The return of normal sleep patterns after a hypnotic is discontinued
    4. The decrease in the amount of REM sleep that causes increased drowsiness

NCLEX item type: multiple choice
Cognitive skill: interpret

11. After discussing with the patient in scenario #1 the best drugs to use for insomnia, the nurse recognizes the need for further education when the patient makes which statement? *(194)*
    1. "So you are saying that I should take drugs for my insomnia for short periods of time to prevent the side effects."
    2. "I see; if I use a hypnotic prior to going to bed this will help with my insomnia."
    3. "You are right. If I don't start getting better sleep it will start to interfere with my work."
    4. "So you are saying that the best type of drug to use for insomnia is a sedative."

Copyright © 2023 by Elsevier, Inc. All rights reserved.

NCLEX item type: cloze
Cognitive skill: evaluate cues

12. The nurse discusses with the patient in scenario #1 the difference between short-term and chronic insomnia and states that short-term insomnia has the features of _____1_____ and _____1_____ while chronic insomnia has the features of _____2_____ and _____2_____. *(193)*

Choose the most likely options for the information missing from the statements below by selecting from the list of options provided.

Option 1	Option 2
Associated with a psychiatric disorder	Associated with job related changes
Lasting less than 3 weeks	Drowsiness that interferes with daytime functioning
Occurs after only a few days	Lasting longer than one month
Associated with travel across time zones	Associated with illness or anxiety

Objective: Discuss nursing interventions that can be implemented as an alternative to administering a sedative-hypnotic medication.

NCLEX item type: multiple responses
Cognitive skill: application

13. While teaching patients about nonpharmacologic methods to enhance sleep, which statements does the nurse include? *(195) (Select all that apply.)*
    1. "It helps if you exercise during the day, but not near bedtime."
    2. "If you try drinking milk before going to bed it may help with insomnia."
    3. "When you are going to bed at the same time each night be certain to go to bed when you feel the most tired."
    4. "Sometimes eating your heaviest meal of the day about 45 minutes before you plan to go to bed works for insomnia."
    5. "Your sleep environment should be quiet and dark and free from distractions."

NCLEX item type: multiple responses
Cognitive skill: contrast

14. When teaching patients with sleep disturbances, which medications and/or substances does the nurse identify as potentially inducing or aggravating insomnia? *(Select all that apply.) (194-195)*
    1. Alcohol
    2. Caffeine
    3. Nicotine
    4. Benzodiazepines
    5. Anticonvulsants

NCLEX item type: multiple response
Cognitive skill: application

15. The nurse knows that the patient who has complained of insomnia can benefit from which alternative methods of inducing sleep? *(Select all that apply.) (195)*
    1. A limitation of stimulants close to bedtime
    2. Avoiding heavy meals late in the evening
    3. Drinking warm milk and eating crackers as a bedtime snack
    4. Limiting exercise during the day and only within 30 minutes of bedtime
    5. Consuming only decaffeinated beverages close to bedtime

NCLEX item type: multiple choice
Cognitive skill: compare

16. The nurse was reviewing a diet choice made by a patient who was suffering from insomnia. Which choice would be a good alternative to a sedative to use to help induce sleep? *(195)*
    1. Chocolate bar and hot milk
    2. Herbal tea and crackers
    3. Hot black tea and a cookie before bed
    4. Glass of wine and dark chocolate

Scenario #2: During the evening shift the nurse learns that a patient who has indicated that they always have to take a sleeping pill in order to sleep noticed that lately it is not working as effectively.

Objective: Compare the effects of benzodiazepines and nonbenzodiazepines on the central nervous system.

NCLEX item type: multiple response
Cognitive skill: explain

17. The patient in scenario # 2 indicates that they have been on zolpidem (Ambien) for sleep. Which statements does the nurse include when teaching a patient about zolpidem (Ambien) therapy? *(Select all that apply.) (200-201)*
    1. "Ambien is available in different forms like sublingual tablets and oral spray."
    2. "It is recommended that this drug be used for 7 to 10 days then reevaluated.."
    3. "Take the medication about 3 hours before you plan on going to sleep."
    4. "The 'morning hangover' side effect is generally not a problem with this medication."
    5. "Ambien has a short onset of action and it lasts for about 4 hours, so it is used for people who have difficulty getting to sleep."

Copyright © 2023 by Elsevier, Inc. All rights reserved.

NCLEX item type: multiple choice
Cognitive skill: interpret
18. The nurse is reviewing the drug class benzodiaz-epine used for insomnia and knows it works by which mechanism of action? *(196)*
    1. By activating the sleep function of the cerebral cortex
    2. By suppressing REM and stages N1 and N2 sleep patterns
    3. By stimulating the neurotransmitter dopamine that initiates sleep
    4. By binding to receptors that stimulate the re-lease of gamma-aminobutyric acid (GABA)

NCLEX item type: extended multiple response
Cognitive skill: recognize cues
19. The nurse recognizes that nonbenzodiazepines, which include the benzodiazepine receptor agonists (e.g., zaleplon, zolpidem, eszopiclone), have which adverse effect that requires careful monitoring? *(201)* *(Select all that apply.)*
    1. Restlessness
    2. Lightheadedness
    3. Blood dyscrasias
    4. Lethargy
    5. Hepatotoxicity
    6. Impaired coordination
    7. Dulled affect
    8. Confusion
    9. Anxiety

NCLEX item type: multiple response
Cognitive skill: application
20. The nurse explains to the patient in scenario #2 what the therapeutic outcomes of benzodiazepine therapy include. Which statements by the nurse need to be corrected? *(Select all that apply.)* *(196)*
    1. "Benzodiazepine therapy is used to produce mild sedation."
    2. "Benzodiazepine therapy is used short-term to produce sleep."
    3. "Benzodiazepine therapy is used to manage migraine headaches."
    4. "Benzodiazepine therapy is used to induce preoperative sedation with amnesia."
    5. "Benzodiazepine therapy is used to increase the amount of REM sleep."

Objective: Identify the antidote drug used for the management of benzodiazepine overdose.
NCLEX item type: multiple choice
Cognitive skill: knowledge
21. A nurse was caring for the patient in scenario #1 who was admitted for benzodiazepine overdose after taking over 20 lorazepam (Ativan) tablets. The nurse expects which medication to be prescribed for the treatment of the overdose? *(196)*
    1. quazepam (Doral)
    2. flumazenil
    3. triazolam (Halcion)
    4. eszopiclone (Lunesta)

NCLEX item type: multiple response
Cognitive skill: interpret
22. The nurse is aware that any rapid discontinuance of benzodiazepines after long-term use may result in symptoms similar to those of alcohol withdrawal, and include which symptoms? *(Select all that apply.)* *(198)*
    1. Delirium
    2. Headaches
    3. Weakness
    4. Anxiety
    5. Grand mal seizures

Objective: Identify laboratory tests that should be monitored when benzodiazepines are administered for an extended period.
NCLEX item type: extended multiple response
Cognitive skill: recognize cues
23. Since one of the common adverse effects of benzodi-azepines is blood dyscrasias, the nurse will monitor which lab values? *(Select all that apply.)* *(198)*
    1. Bilirubin
    2. Red blood cells
    3. Electrolytes
    4. Alkaline phosphatase
    5. White blood cells with differential
    6. Platelets
    7. Prothrombin time

NCLEX item type: multiple response
Cognitive skill: application
24. The nurse will monitor the patient when taking benzodiazepines for symptoms of hepatotoxicity which include anorexia, nausea, vomiting, jaundice, hepatomegaly, splenomegaly, and abnormal liver function tests. Laboratory results that are moni-tored for abnormal liver function tests include what results? *(Select all that apply.)* *(198)*
    1. Bilirubin
    2. Platelets
    3. Alkaline phosphatase
    4. Aspartate aminotransferase [AST]
    5. Alanine aminotransferase [ALT]

NCLEX item type: multiple choice
Cognitive skill: predict
25. The nurse explains to a female patient that a preg-nancy test should be ordered when started on a benzodiazepine, since these agents may have which effect? *(198)*
    1. The morning hangover effect will last all day.
    2. The withdrawal symptoms are worse for preg-nant mothers.
    3. There is an increased incidence of maternal deaths after use of these drugs.
    4. There is an increased incidence of birth defects because these agents cross the placenta.

Copyright © 2023 by Elsevier, Inc. All rights reserved.

Drugs Used to Treat Neurodegenerative Disorders

chapter

14

Answer Key: Textbook page references are provided as a guide for answering these questions. A complete answer key is provided to your instructor.

MATCHING
Match the definition to the terminology used in neurodegenerative disorders.

Definition

1. _____ a lack of movement

2. _____ quick, short steps that may be forward or backward unintentionally

3. _____ a diffuse rose-colored mottling of the skin

4. _____ a chronic, progressive disorder of the central nervous system causing movement disorders

5. _____ a progressive neurodegenerative disease causing cognitive dysfunction

6. _____ a shaking often observed in the hands, and may involve the jaws, lips, and tongue

7. _____ an impairment of the ability to perform voluntary movement

Neurodegenerative terminology

a. Parkinson disease
b. Alzheimer disease
c. dyskinesia
d. akinesia
e. tremors
f. livedo reticularis
g. propulsive, uncontrolled movement

REVIEW QUESTIONS
Scenario #1: A 57-year-old patient who was diagnosed with Parkinson disease is admitted to an inpatient unit to regulate his medications.

Objective: Identify the signs and symptoms of Parkinson disease
NCLEX item type: multiple response
Cognitive skill: application

8. The nurse caring for the patient in scenario #1 expects to see the patient exhibit symptoms that include difficulty walking and possibly stooped posture, as well as what other symptoms? *(Select all that apply.)* *(204)*
   1. Muscle tremors
   2. Urinary retention
   3. Muscle weakness with rigidity
   4. Posture and equilibrium changes
   5. Slowness of movement in performing daily activities

NCLEX item type: multiple choice
Cognitive skill: comprehension
9. The nurse understands that Parkinson disease is caused by a deterioration of what? *(204)*
   1. The levodopa receptors
   2. The dopaminergic neurons
   3. The cholinergic fibers
   4. The acetylcholine neurons

NCLEX item type: multiple response
Cognitive skill: application
10. The nurse recognizes that although Parkinson disease is primarily considered a disease that affects the patient's ability to walk, it also has nonmotor symptoms such as what? *(Select all that apply.)* *(204)*
   1. Depression
   2. Nocturnal sleep disturbances
   3. Constipation
   4. Bladder incontinence
   5. Chronic fatigue

Copyright © 2023 by Elsevier, Inc. All rights reserved.

NCLEX item type: multiple choice
Cognitive skill: knowledge

11. Which symptom of Parkinson disease is manifested as extremely slow body movements that may eventually progress to a total lack of movement? *(206)*
    1. Akinesia
    2. Dyskinesia
    3. Bradykinesia
    4. Propulsive movement

Objective: Identify the neurotransmitter that is found in excess and the neurotransmitter that is deficient in people with parkinsonism

NCLEX item type: multiple choice
Cognitive skill: relate

12. The nurse provided education for the patient in the scenario with Parkinson disease on what causes their symptoms and explained that which neurotransmitter is deficient? *(204)*
    1. "Your symptoms of this disease are causes by the destruction of the neurons that produce norepinephrine."
    2. "Your symptoms of this disease are causes by the destruction of the neurons that produce dopamine."
    3. "Your symptoms of this disease are causes by the destruction of the neurons that produce serotonin."
    4. "Your symptoms of this disease are causes by the destruction of the neurons that produce acetylcholine."

NCLEX item type: multiple choice
Cognitive skill: knowledge

13. The nurse provided education for the patient in the scenario with Parkinson disease on what causes the symptoms and explained that which neurotransmitter is in excess? *(204)*
    1. "Your symptoms are caused by an excess of the neurotransmitter serotonin."
    2. "Your symptoms are caused by an excess of the neurotransmitter norepinephrine."
    3. "Your symptoms are caused by an excess of the neurotransmitter acetylcholine."
    4. "Your symptoms are caused by an excess of the neurotransmitter dopamine."

NCLEX item type: multiple response
Cognitive skill: application

14. There are several causes for secondary parkinsonism that the nurse recalls as what? *(Select all that apply.)* *(205)*
    1. Tumors
    2. Hereditary
    3. Intracranial infections
    4. Head trauma
    5. Unknown causes

Objective: Discuss the action of carbidopa levodopa, and dopamine agonists in Parkinson disease

NCLEX item type: multiple choice
Cognitive skill: interpret

15. The patient in scenario #1 was previously controlled on carbidopa-levodopa and now was finding that the effects were wearing off. The nurse explained to the patient what the major action of the drug carbidopa does when combined with levodopa. Which statement by the nurse is correct? *(211)*
    1. "Carbidopa when combined with levodopa will reduce the production of dopamine."
    2. "Carbidopa when combined with levodopa will reduce the metabolism of levodopa."
    3. "Carbidopa when combined with levodopa will increase the metabolism of levodopa."
    4. "Carbidopa when combined with levodopa will allow more levodopa to be absorbed."

NCLEX item type: multiple choice
Cognitive skill: explain

16. The nurse explains to the patient in scenario # 1 that the drugs carbidopa-levodopa (Sinemet) must be given in combination because of which effect? *(211)*
    1. Levodopa has no effect when used alone.
    2. Carbidopa has no effect when used alone.
    3. Levodopa is used to reduce the dose of carbidopa required.
    4. Carbidopa is used to increase the dose of levodopa required.

NCLEX item type: multiple choice
Cognitive skill: knowledge

17. Generally, patients with Parkinson disease will be treated with carbidopa-levodopa, but the drug's effect gradually wears off by which timeframe? *(211)*
    1. In 12-24 months
    2. In 3-5 years
    3. In 1-2 years
    4. In 6-8 months

NCLEX item type: multiple response
Cognitive skill: take action

18. What are the nursing considerations for patients on apomorphine (Apokyn) therapy? *(Select all that apply.)* *(215)*
    1. Do not administer apomorphine intravenously.
    2. Calculate apomorphine dose based on milligrams.
    3. Administer prochlorperazine for nausea associated with apomorphine therapy.
    4. Assess patients on apomorphine therapy for orthostatic hypotension.
    5. Assess patients receiving apomorphine therapy for sudden sleep attacks.

Copyright © 2023 by Elsevier, Inc. All rights reserved.

NCLEX item type: multiple choice
Cognitive skill: contrast

19. The nurse recognizes which classification of drugs is used to treat parkinsonism by reducing the metabolism of dopamine in the brain? *(209)*
    1. COMT inhibitors
    2. Anticholinergic agents
    3. Monoamine oxidase type B inhibitors
    4. Selective serotonin reuptake inhibitors

Objective: Explain the action of entacapone, opicapone, and of the monoamine oxidase inhibitors (selegiline, safinamide, and rasagiline) as it relates to the treatment of Parkinson disease

NCLEX item type: multiple choice
Cognitive skill: illustrate

20. The nurse reviews the major action of the drug entacapone (Comtan), which is a COMT inhibitor and noted it works how? *(220)*
    1. By increasing the absorption of dopamine
    2. By slowing the progression of deterioration of dopaminergic nerve cells
    3. By increasing the adverse dopaminergic effects of levodopa
    4. By reducing the destruction of dopamine in the peripheral tissues

NCLEX item type: multiple choice
Cognitive skill: knowledge

21. Active metabolites of selegiline (Eldepryl), when swallowed, are amphetamines that cause cardiovascular and psychiatric adverse effects. To avoid this effect, how does the nurse administer the drug? *(209)*
    1. A rectal suppository
    2. A subcutaneous injection
    3. An orally disintegrating tablet
    4. An intradermal injection

NCLEX item type: multiple choice
Cognitive skill: relate

22. When patients start on monoamine oxidase type B inhibitor therapy in conjunction with carbidopa-levodopa (Sinemet), the dosages of Sinemet can be titrated downward starting when? *(210)*
    1. After month 4 or 5 of therapy
    2. After month 2 or 3 of therapy
    3. After week 2 or 3 of therapy
    4. After day 2 or 3 of therapy

NCLEX item type: cloze
Cognitive skill: recognize cues

23. The nurse explains to the patient with Parkinson's disease that the drug _____1_____ reduces the destruction of dopamine in the peripheral tissues, allowing significantly more _____2_____ to reach the brain to eliminate the symptoms of parkinsonism? *(220)*

Choose the most likely options for the information missing from the statements below by selecting from the list of options provided.

Option 1	Option 2
Apomorphine (Apokyn)	Norepinephrine
Ropinirole (Requip)	Acetylcholine
Entacapone (Comtan)	Epinephrine
Selegiline (Eldepryl)	Dopamine

Objective: Discuss the specific symptoms that should show improvement when anticholinergic agents are administered to a patient with Parkinson disease

NCLEX item type: multiple response
Cognitive skill: application

24. What are the therapeutic outcomes that the nurse can expect for a patient after being treated for Parkinson disease with anticholinergic agents? *(Select all that apply.) (221)*
    1. Improvement in their gait and posture
    2. Decreased depression level and improved mood
    3. Improvement in speech pattern
    4. Decrease in drooling
    5. Decrease in the severity of the tremors

NCLEX item type: multiple choice
Cognitive skill: explain

25. The nurse explains to the patient in scenario #1 that the main reason anticholinergic agents are prescribed for patients with parkinsonism is because these agents will do what? *(221)*
    1. Decrease the absorption of acetylcholine
    2. Increase the absorption of dopamine
    3. Reduce hyperstimulation caused by the excess amount of acetylcholine
    4. Prevent the adverse effect of orthostatic hypotension

Copyright © 2023 by Elsevier, Inc. All rights reserved.

NCLEX item type: multiple choice
Cognitive skill: comprehension

26. What nursing assessments are needed for patients who are starting on carbidopa-levodopa therapy? *(221)*
    1. Perform a baseline assessment using UPDRS.
    2. Plan to perform a baseline assessment every 3 months while on the drug.
    3. Observe for the drug's therapeutic effect to occur within 2 weeks of therapy.
    4. Anticipate the patient developing involuntary movement such as bobbing within 2 weeks of therapy.

NCLEX item type: extended multiple response
Cognitive skill: recognize cues

27. The nurse reviewed the adverse effects of anticholinergic agents and identifies which ones? *(Select all that apply.)* *(222)*
    1. Dry mouth
    2. Diarrhea
    3. Runny nose
    4. Dry nose
    5. Constipation
    6. Drooling
    7. Urinary retention
    8. Tremors

Scenario #2: An Alzheimer patient was brought into the clinic by their family because their behavior was becoming to hard to manage. The patient was becoming aggressive toward the family and was refusing to comply when directed to participate in regular ADLs.

Objective: Explain the action of the agents used in the treatment of Alzheimer's disease
NCLEX item type: multiple choice
Cognitive skill: compare

28. The nurse reviews the primary action of donepezil (Aricept) prior to administration and understands that this drug will effect what? *(224)*
    1. It prevents the loss of cholinergic neurons.
    2. It allows norepinephrine to accumulate at the neuron synapses.
    3. It inhibits acetylcholinesterase, the enzyme that breaks down acetylcholine.

    4. It activates acetylcholinesterase, the enzyme that breaks down acetylcholine.

NCLEX item type: multiple choice
Cognitive skill: explain

29. The nurse is teaching the patient's caregiver in scenario #2 about the primary therapeutic outcome of memantine (Namenda). Which statement by the nurse is correct? *(225)*
    1. "We expect that the memantine will enhance muscle tone."
    2. "We can expect an improvement of cognitive skills with memantine."
    3. "We have found that there is an improvement of mobility and coordination with memantine."
    4. "We use memantine to prevent or slow the degeneration of the neurons that occurs in Alzheimer's disease."

NCLEX item type: multiple response
Cognitive skill: application

30. Which statements does the nurse include when teaching a patient and family about donepezil (Aricept)? *(Select all that apply.)* *(224)*
    1. "Donepezil must be taken on an empty stomach."
    2. "This drug will prevent your disease from getting worse."
    3. "Notify your healthcare provider if your pulse is fewer than 60 beats per minute."
    4. "Discontinue the drug if you develop diarrhea early in the treatment program."
    5. "You may feel a little nauseated when first taking this medication, but this usually subsides after 2–3 weeks of therapy."

Copyright © 2023 by Elsevier, Inc. All rights reserved.

Drugs Used for Anxiety Disorders

chapter

15

Answer Key: Textbook page references are provided as a guide for answering these questions. A complete answer key is provided to your instructor.

MATCHING

Match the definition on the right with the term on the left.

Term

1. _____ generalized anxiety disorder
2. _____ panic attack
3. _____ anxiolytics
4. _____ obsessive-compulsive disorder
5. _____ phobias

Definition

a. an abrupt surge of intense fear or intense discomfort
b. excessive and unrealistic worry about two or more life circumstances
c. recurrent thoughts or actions that cause significant distress and interfere with normal functioning
d. irrational fears of specific objects, activities, or situations
e. antianxiety medications

REVIEW QUESTIONS

Scenario #1: A 58-year-old patient was admitted for further evaluation of bizarre behavior manifested as loud, rapid talking; pacing; and wringing of the hands. Relatives have attempted to calm the patient with no effect, and they brought the patient to urgent care for consultation.

Objective: Compare and contrast the differences among generalized anxiety disorder, panic disorder, phobias, and obsessive-compulsive disorder

NCLEX item type: multiple choice
Cognitive skill: compare

6. The nurse is caring for a patient with the irrational fear of a having their blood drawn, and can even recognize the fear as exaggerated or unrealistic. Which statement by the nurse explains this behavior? *(229)*
   1. "People have fears of all kinds of situations and activities that are irrational but feel very real called phobias."
   2. "This fear occurs suddenly and overwhelms people and is often relapsing called a panic disorder."
   3. "When people become irrational about certain situations this can trigger a generalized anxiety disorder."
   4. "Obsessive-compulsive behavior is performed to decrease anxiety that people feel and is a very complex condition."

NCLEX item type: multiple response
Cognitive skill: application

7. The nurse monitors the patient in scenario #1 who demonstrates psychomotor symptoms of anxiety for physiologic signs of anxiety. ? *(Select all that apply.) (228)*
   1. Tachycardia
   2. Decreased energy
   3. Palpitations
   4. Increased urination
   5. Sweating

NCLEX item type: multiple choice
Cognitive skill: comprehension

8. When patients have unwanted thoughts, ideas, images, or an urge that the patient recognizes as time-consuming and senseless but repeatedly intrudes into the consciousness despite attempts to ignore, prevent, or counteract it, the patient is said to be experiencing what? *(229)*
   1. A phobia
   2. A panic disorder
   3. A generalized anxiety disorder
   4. An obsessive-compulsive disorder

Copyright © 2023 by Elsevier, Inc. All rights reserved.

Objective: Describe the essential components included in a baseline assessment of a patient's mental status

NCLEX item type: multiple choice
Cognitive skill: interpret

9. In scenario #1, the urgent care nurse will regularly assess the patient for which symptoms to determine if acute hospitalization is indicated? *(230)*
   1. Patient is complaining of nausea and refuses breakfast.
   2. Patient appears to be at risk for harming themself or others.
   3. Patient has a clean and neat appearance, and the ability to perform self-care.
   4. Patient demonstrates a stooped or slumped posture, and is alert and oriented.

NCLEX item type: multiple choice
Cognitive skill: knowledge

10. Why is it important for the nurse to identify events that trigger anxiety in patients? *(230)*
    1. To be aware of what to avoid talking about with the patient
    2. To reintroduce the trigger in a controlled environment and cure the patient of their anxiety
    3. To question the validity of the anxiety to help the patient see how foolish it is
    4. To help the patient to reduce anxiety or cope more adaptively with stressors

NCLEX item type: multiple response
Cognitive skill: application

11. The nurse is taking care of the patient in scenario #1 and performs a baseline mental status assessment, which will include asking the patient to describe what normal patterns? *(Select all that apply.)* *(231)*
    1. Sleep
    2. Weight gains or losses
    3. Family interactions
    4. Psychomotor functions
    5. Obsessions or compulsions

Scenario #2: A patient with generalized anxiety disorder treated with oxazepam came to the outpatient clinic for a checkup and medication review.

Objective: Discuss the drug therapy used to treat anxiety disorders

NCLEX item type: multiple response
Cognitive skill: compare

12. The nurse reviewed which drug classes used to treat patients with anxiety disorders? *(Select all that apply.)* *(232-235)*
    1. Benzodiazepines
    2. Azaspirones
    3. Calcium channel blockers
    4. Selective serotonin reuptake inhibitors (SSRIs)
    5. Monoamine oxidase type B inhibitors

NCLEX item type: extended multiple response
Cognitive skill: recognize cues

13. The nurse educates the patient who is started on hydroxyzine therapy used as a mild tranquilizer for psychiatric conditions. What other uses does hydroxyzine have? *(Select all that apply.)* *(235)*
    1. As an antihistamine for mild allergies
    2. As an antiemetic for nausea
    3. As an antianxiety for agitation
    4. As an antidote for excess dopamine
    5. As an antacid for reflux disease
    6. As an antipruritic agent to relieve itching
    7. As an antiepileptic for seizures

NCLEX item type: multiple choice
Cognitive skill: interpret

14. When explaining why patients who experience anxiety with other conditions are treated with benzodiazepine therapy the nurse made which statement that needed to be corrected? *(232)*
    1. "Benzodiazepines are used because they are consistently effective."
    2. "Patients who develop anxiety reactions to recent events and treatable medical illnesses will respond most readily with a reduction in anxiety when treated with benzodiazepines."
    3. "Benzodiazepines are used because there is less potential for abuse than other antianxiety agents."
    4. "In patients with reduced hepatic function oxazepam may not be appropriate because of its short duration of action."

NCLEX item type: multiple choice
Cognitive skill: compare

15. The benzodiazepine drug monograph lists hepatotoxicity as a serious adverse effect. Which laboratory tests does the nurse monitor to assess this? *(234)*
    1. Creatinine, creatinine clearance, and blood urea nitrogen (BUN)
    2. Hematocrit, ferritin, and prothrombin time
    3. Aspartate aminotransferase (AST), alanine aminotransferase (ALT), and alkaline phosphatase
    4. Potassium, sodium, chloride and magnesium

NCLEX item type: multiple choice
Cognitive skill: relate

16. What information does the nurse include during teaching for the patient in scenario #2 who is taking antianxiety therapy? *(233-234)*
    1. "You may take this medication while operating machinery."
    2. "Therapeutic effects of the drug take 4–6 weeks to occur."
    3. "When discontinuing the medication, there is no need to reduce the dose gradually."
    4. "Notify your healthcare provider if hangover symptoms persist, because the dose may need to be reduced or the medication changed."

Copyright © 2023 by Elsevier, Inc. All rights reserved.

Objective: Identify adverse effects that may result from drug therapy used to treat anxiety

NCLEX item type: multiple choice

Cognitive skill: knowledge

17. Nurses need to teach patients taking hydroxyzine therapy for anxiety to report which symptoms that should be monitored? *(236)*
    1. Dry mouth
    2. Slurred speech and dizziness
    3. Reduction in anxiety
    4. Constipation

NCLEX item type: multiple response

Cognitive skill: evaluate outcomes

18. The nursing implications for buspirone therapy include watching for adverse effects of the drug which include which symptoms? *(Select all that apply.)* *(234)*
    1. Dizziness and insomnia
    2. Orthostatic hypotension
    3. Sedation and lethargy
    4. Nervousness and drowsiness
    5. Restless leg syndrome

NCLEX item type: multiple response

Cognitive skill: application

19. The nurse reviewed the medication list of a patient taking benzodiazepines for potential drug interactions. Which drugs may increase the toxic effects of benzodiazepines? *(Select all that apply.)* *(234)*
    1. Antihistamines
    2. Opioids
    3. Probenecid
    4. Rifampin
    5. Valproic acid

Objective: Discuss psychologic and physiologic drug dependence

NCLEX item type: multiple response

Cognitive skill: take action

20. When a patient is experiencing withdrawal symptoms from long-term use of benzodiazepines, the nurse assesses for which effect ? *(Select all that apply.)* *(233)*
    1. Weakness
    2. Anxiety
    3. Delirium
    4. Decreased heart rate
    5. Tonic-clonic seizures

NCLEX item type: multiple choice

Cognitive skill: knowledge

21. The nurse is assessing a patient before administering buspirone. Which finding would the nurse call the healthcare provider about to determine the appropriateness of the drug? *(234)*
    1. Slurred speech
    2. Insomnia
    3. Nervousness
    4. Dizziness

NCLEX item type: cloze

Cognitive skill: recognize cues

22. The nurse understands that the drug _____1_____ taken for anxiety may cause psychologic and physiologic dependence. *(233)*

Choose the most likely option for the information missing from the statements below by selecting from the list of options provided:

Option 1
Hydroxyzine
Diazepam
Buspirone
Fluvoxamine

Copyright © 2023 by Elsevier, Inc. All rights reserved.

Drugs Used for Depressive and Bipolar Disorders

chapter

16

Answer Key: Textbook page references are provided as a guide for answering these questions. A complete answer key is provided to your instructor.

MATCHING

Match the definition on the right with the term on the left.

Term

1. _____ depression
2. _____ mania
3. _____ cyclothymia
4. _____ euphoria
5. _____ grandiose delusions
6. _____ dysthymia
7. _____ labile mood
8. _____ suicidal ideation

Definition

a. the delusion that one has great talents or special powers
b. a milder form of bipolar illness characterized by episodes of depression and hypomania
c. a rapid shift in mood toward anger and irritability
d. a persistent, reduced ability to experience pleasure in life's usual activities
e. a heightened mood
f. thoughts about killing oneself
g. a mood disturbance characterized by elation and euphoria
h. a chronic form of depression with ongoing symptoms lasting for at least 2 years

REVIEW QUESTIONS

Scenario #1: A 78-year-old patient came into the clinic describing symptoms of feeling blue, experiencing insomnia, and having a lack of motivation to do daily activities, which has been increasing in occurrence for the last several months.

Objective: Describe the essential components of the baseline assessment of a patient with depression or bipolar disorder

NCLEX item type: multiple response
Cognitive skill: application

9. The nurse is assessing the patient in scenario #1 for characteristic symptoms found in a person experiencing depression. What are some cognitive symptoms the nurse is looking for? *(Select all that apply.)* *(239)*
    1. Poor memory of recent events
    2. Slowed thinking
    3. Extreme changes in mood
    4. Inability to concentrate
    5. Increase in appetite

NCLEX item type: multiple response
Cognitive skill: evaluate

10. What features of depression does the patient in scenario #1 exhibit that indicate to the nurse this might be the issue? *(239)* *(Select all that apply.)*
    1. Feeling blue
    2. Recent weight gain
    3. Lack of motivation
    4. Labile mood
    5. Insomnia

NCLEX item type: multiple response
Cognitive skill: application

11. The nurse is assessing a patient who is being started on imipramine for depression and is reviewing the basic components of the assessment for mood disorders, which include asking the patient about their history of what factors? *(Select all that apply.)* *(252)*
    1. Hygiene habits
    2. Thoughts of death
    3. Job expectation
    4. Interpersonal relationships
    5. History of mood disorders

Copyright © 2023 by Elsevier, Inc. All rights reserved.

NCLEX item type: drop and drag
Cognitive skill: analyze cues
12. The nurse reviewed the symptoms associated with depression and bipolar disorders.

Using an arrow, draw a line from the characteristic of the disorder to the definition. *(239-240)*

Characteristics	Definition
Episodes of depression and hypomania	Depression (cognitive symptoms)
Slowed thinking, confusion, and poor memory	Labile mood
Pacing, hand-wringing, and outbursts of shouting	Bipolar disorder
Episodes of mania and depression separated by intervals without mood disturbances	Depression (psychomotor symptoms)
Rapid shits toward anger an irritability	Cyclothymia

NCLEX item type: cloze
Cognitive skill: recognize cues
13. The nurse recognizes the symptoms of
_____1_____ in patients with bipolar disorder which may include _____2_____
and _____2_____. *(239-240)*

Choose the most likely options for the information missing from the statements below by selecting from the list of options provided.

Option 1	Option 2
Acute mania	Increased need for sleep
Cyclothymia	Heightened mood (euphoria)
Labile mood	Flight of ideas
Hypomania	Feeling sad

NCLEX item type: multiple choice
Cognitive skill: comprehension
14. Nurses know that when patients experience the manic phase of bipolar disorder they generally do what? *(240)*
1. Develop a stable mood during this phase
2. Will not develop psychotic symptoms
3. Tend to have suicidal ideation
4. Will not recognize the symptoms of illness in themselves

Objective: Identify the premedication assessments that are necessary before the administration of monoamine oxidase inhibitors (MAOIs), selective serotonin reuptake inhibitors (SSRIs), serotonin-norepinephrine reuptake inhibitors (SNRIs), tricyclic antidepressants (TCAs), and antimanic agents

NCLEX item type: multiple choice
Cognitive skill: knowledge
15. When patients experience the physiologic manifestations of depression such as sleep disturbance, change in appetite, loss of energy, fatigue, or palpitations, they can expect to have some relief from these symptoms after starting on a monoamine oxidase inhibitor (MOAI) antidepressant within what timeframe? *(245)*
1. Within the first three doses of starting therapy
2. After the second day of starting therapy
3. Within 2–4 weeks of starting therapy
4. After the sixth week of starting therapy

NCLEX item type: multiple response
Cognitive skill: application
16. What are important premedication assessments will the nurse perform when caring for patients starting on selective serotonin reuptake inhibitors (SSRIs)? *(Select all that apply.)* *(249)*
1. Note any GI symptoms present before starting therapy
2. Obtain the patient's baseline blood pressure
3. Check the patient's lab values for liver enzymes
4. Determine the patient's primary insurance payer
5. Obtain the patient's baseline weight and measure weight weekly
6. Monitor the patient's hearing prior to administration

NCLEX item type: grid/matrix
Cognitive skill: analysis cues
17. The nurse was performing a premedication assessment on a patient who was being started on a serotonin-norepinephrine reuptake inhibitors (SNRIs). Indicate with an X the significant findings that need to be reported and the findings the non-essential findings. *(251)*

	Essential findings	Nonessential findings
Daily use of alcohol		
Good appetite		
Elevated creatinine levels		
Hypertension		
Hyperthyroidism		

Copyright © 2023 by Elsevier, Inc. All rights reserved.

NCLEX item type: multiple response
Cognitive skill: take action

18. The premedication assessment that nurses perform for TCAs includes which nursing intervention? *(Select all that apply.) (252)*
    1. Checking for a history of seizures
    2. Obtaining the patient's height and weight
    3. Determining if there is any history of dysrhythmias
    4. Taking the patient's blood pressure and reporting hypotension
    5. Noting constituency of the patient's stools to watch for constipation

NCLEX item type: multiple response
Cognitive skill: analyze

19. The medication assessment that nurses perform for lithium, an antimanic agent includes which nursing intervention? *(Select all that apply.) (258)*
    1. Weighing the patient weekly
    2. Obtaining baseline blood pressures supine, and standing
    3. Administering lithium on an empty stomach
    4. Obtaining laboratory tests such as electrolytes, blood glucose, and blood urea nitrogen (BUN)
    5. Monitoring lithium levels once or twice weekly during the start of therapy

Objective: Describe the common adverse effects that may develop for patients who are taking MAOIs

NCLEX item type: multiple response
Cognitive skill: application

20. When patients are taking MAOIs, the nurse needs to include which instructions for patients? *(Select all that apply.) (245, 248)*
    1. How to limit tyramine-containing foods in their diet
    2. The importance of not discontinuing the drug abruptly
    3. To avoid taking the divided dose later than 8 PM
    4. Dividing the dose to prevent drug-induced insomnia
    5. Avoiding the drugs known to cause drug interactions

NCLEX item type: multiple choice
Cognitive skill: knowledge

21. When patients are taking the MAOI drug selegiline (Emsam), the nurse needs to assess for which adverse effect? *(248)*
    1. Vomiting and diarrhea
    2. Drowsiness and sedation
    3. Therapeutic serum levels
    4. Increased salivation

NCLEX item type: multiple choice
Cognitive skill: interpret

22. The nurse was instructing a diabetic patient who was starting on the MAOI isocarboxazid (Marplan) regarding precautions to use, and realized further education was needed after the patient made which statement? *(245)*
    1. "Since I have to take insulin, I will need to adjust my doses while I take this drug."
    2. "As I understand it, I can stop taking my insulin since this drug will cause hypoglycemia."
    3. "I get it; I need to carefully monitor my blood sugar while I am on this drug."
    4. "I will need to carefully determine what foods I can eat while on this drug."

Objective: Describe the common adverse effects that may develop for patients who are taking SSRIs and SNRIs

NCLEX item type: multiple choice
Cognitive skill: analyze

23. The nurse instructed the patient in scenario #1 who is starting on escitalopram (Lexapro) on the adverse effects, and knows that SSRIs and SNRIs have the same common adverse effects. Which statement by the patient indicates further teaching is needed? *(249-250)*
    1. "I will take this tablet once a day, but it may make me drowsy. Luckily I no longer need to drive for a living."
    2. "So you say that if I take this med with food it should not cause me to feel nauseated."
    3. "As I understand it, I should avoid taking this at night since it may cause insomnia."
    4. "I will watch for constipation while on this drug since that is one of the side effects."

NCLEX item type: multiple response
Cognitive skill: application

24. What do nurses need to assess for in patients prior to starting therapy with the SNRI duloxetine (Cymbalta)? *(Select all that apply.) (251)*
    1. GI symptoms
    2. Glaucoma
    3. Insomnia
    4. Hypertension
    5. Thyroid disorders

Copyright © 2023 by Elsevier, Inc. All rights reserved.

NCLEX item type: multiple choice
Cognitive skill: explain
25. The nurse teaching the patient in scenario #1 about how important medication safety is with SSRIs includes which statement in the education? *(249)*
    1. "It is important to weigh yourself on a weekly basis."
    2. "When you are taking this medication you need to be careful about avoiding foods containing tyramine."
    3. "These drugs may cause serotonin syndrome due to the excess accumulation of serotonin in your system, which is uncommon but potentially fatal."
    4. "You need to keep track of how well you are feeling and that your depression improves."

Objective: Describe the common adverse effects that may develop for patients who are taking TCAs
NCLEX item type: multiple choice
Cognitive skill: knowledge
26. When patients are taking TCAs for depression, what is the most important baseline parameter the nurse needs to assess? *(252)*
    1. Pulse oximetry
    2. Weight
    3. Temperature
    4. Blood pressure in supine and sitting positions
NCLEX item type: multiple response
Cognitive skill: application
27. Primary outcomes expected from TCAs include elevated mood and reduction of symptoms of depression, and TCAs can also be used for the treatment of which conditions? *(Select all that apply.)* *(252)*
    1. Anxiety
    2. Glaucoma
    3. Phantom limb pain
    4. Enuresis in children
    5. Obsessive-compulsive disorders
NCLEX item type: multiple response
Cognitive skill: compare
28. When patients are taking the TCA drug desipramine (Norpramin) the nurse needs to assess for which common adverse effect? *(252)*
    1. Orthostatic hypotension
    2. Blurred vision
    3. Hearing loss
    4. Parkinsonian symptoms
    5. Constipation

Scenario #2: A patient admitted to the psychiatric wing of the hospital was newly diagnosed with bipolar disorder. The patient subsequently started on lithium to control the symptoms and the nurse will education the patient on precautions to take while on lithium.

Objective: Describe the common adverse effects that may develop for patients who are taking lithium
NCLEX item type: multiple choice
Cognitive skill: knowledge
29. The nurse teaching the patient in scenario #2 about lithium discussed the adverse effects. Which statement does the nurse include in the education? *(258)*
    1. "While you are taking lithium you will need to limit your fluid intake."
    2. "If you get nausea or abdominal cramps, you can take lithium with food."
    3. "You may develop hand tremors, but they will go away in a few days."
    4. "If you develop excessive urination, this is a sign of toxicity and you need to discontinue therapy."
NCLEX item type: multiple response
Cognitive skill: application
30. When the antimanic agent lithium is used for patients with bipolar disorder, the nurse educates the patient and family on which ways to prevent toxicity? *(Select all that apply.)* *(258)*
    1. "Lithium may to be taken with food or milk."
    2. "Report any persistent vomiting or profuse diarrhea, as this may imply toxicity."
    3. "You will need to maintain a normal dietary intake of sodium with adequate water."
    4. "You will need to monitor your lithium levels once or twice weekly during the start of this therapy."
    5. "Report weight gain and feeling of progressive fatigue, as these may indicate toxicity."

Copyright © 2023 by Elsevier, Inc. All rights reserved.

Drugs Used for Psychoses

Answer Key: Textbook page references are provided as a guide for answering these questions. A complete answer key is provided to your instructor.

MATCHING
Match the term on the right with the definition on the left.

Definition

1. _____ spasmodic movements of muscle groups

2. _____ a syndrome of persistent and involuntary hyperkinetic abnormal movements

3. _____ tremors, muscle rigidity, mask-like expressions, shuffling gait, and loss or weakness of motor function

4. _____ a syndrome of anxiety and restlessness, and associated pacing, rocking, and an inability to sit or stand in one place for extended periods

5. _____ term that applies to someone who is out of touch with reality

6. _____ adverse effects of antipsychotic medications associated with nonadherence to therapy

7. _____ false sensory perceptions, experienced as real to the patient

Term

a. pseudoparkinsonian symptoms
b. hallucinations
c. tardive dyskinesia
d. akathisia
e. extrapyramidal symptoms
f. dystonias
g. psychosis

REVIEW QUESTIONS

Scenario: A 45-year-old male patient was admitted to the inpatient psychiatric unit for further evaluation and treatment after he was found by his family to be babbling incoherently and rapidly pacing in his apartment. He has a history of schizoid affective disorder and had not taken his medications lately.

Objective: Identify the signs and symptoms of psychotic behavior.
NCLEX item type: multiple response
Cognitive skill: application
8. The nurse admitting the patient in the scenario who is said to be suffering from psychosis recognizes which of these symptoms of psychotic behavior? *(Select all that apply.) (262)*
   1. Insomnia
   2. Delusions
   3. Hallucinations
   4. Orthostatic hypotension
   5. Disorganized thinking

NCLEX item type: multiple choice
Cognitive skill: comprehension
9. A patient in the emergency department tells the nurse that they are the creator of the universe. What does the nurse suspect that this patient is experiencing? *(262)*
   1. Delusions
   2. Hallucinations
   3. Flight of ideas
   4. Disorganized behavior

NCLEX item type: multiple response
Cognitive skill: application
10. Target symptoms are critical monitoring parameters used to assess changes in the patient's status and their response to medications. Which are examples of target symptoms? *(Select all that apply.) (263)*
   1. Weight gain
   2. Loose associations
   3. Substance abuse
   4. Frequency and type of agitation
   5. Degree of suspiciousness

Copyright © 2023 by Elsevier, Inc. All rights reserved.

Objective: Describe the major indications for the use of antipsychotic agents.
NCLEX item type: multiple choice
Cognitive skill: analyze

11. The nurse discussed with the patient's family in the scenario about the indications for the use of antipsychotic agents. Which statement by the nurse needs to be corrected? *(262-263)*
    1. "Psychotic disorders are extremely complex illnesses and some require several months before a final diagnosis is determined."
    2. "Psychotic symptoms are common in patients with mood disorders such as major depression and biplolar disorders."
    3. "Nonpharmacologic interventions generally do not benefit patients with psychoses so drug therapy is more important."
    4. "Before initiating therapy treatment goals need to be determined as well as level of functioning."

NCLEX item type: multiple response
Cognitive skill: application

12. The nurse explains to the patient in the scenario the need to continue on their prescribed medications. An indication for being on antipsychotic agents would be to help control psychotic symptoms common with which mood disorders? *(Select all that apply.)* *(262)*
    1. Anorexia
    2. Schizophrenia
    3. Bipolar disorder
    4. Major depression
    5. Obsessive-compulsive disorder

NCLEX item type: cloze
Cognitive skill: recognize cues

13. The nurse knows that psychotic symptoms can be caused by an underlying illness that needs to be treated along with the psychosis. Examples of these underlying illnesses include _____1_____ and _____1_____ and _____1_____. *(262)*

Choose the most likely options for the information missing from the statements below by selecting from the list of options provided.

Option 1

Infections

Traumatic brain injuries

Metabolic disorders

Strokes

Dementias

Objective: Discuss the antipsychotic medications that are used for the treatment of psychoses.
NCLEX item type: multiple choice
Cognitive skill: interpret

14. The nurse had an order to administer prochlorperazine, a first-generation antipsychotic agent. Prochlorperazine, a phenothiazine is thought to have which mechanism of action? *(272)*
    1. Block serotonin reuptake
    2. Block the serotonin receptors
    3. Block dopamine receptors
    4. Release serotonin at receptor sites

NCLEX item type: multiple choice
Cognitive skill: analyze

15. The patient in the scenario was being started on risperidone, a second-generation or atypical antipsychotic agent. The nurse researched the drugs mechanism of action and found they have which effect? *(272)*
    1. Block serotonin reuptake
    2. Block the dopamine and serotonin receptors
    3. Block dopamine receptors
    4. Release serotonin at receptor sites

NCLEX item type: multiple response
Cognitive skill: classify

16. The nurse reviewed the atypical antipsychotic agents that are most commonly used because they tend to be more effective in relieving negative symptoms. These agents include which medications? *(Select all that apply.)* *(272)*
    1. haloperidol (Haldol)
    2. risperidone (Risperdal)
    3. quetiapine (Seroquel)
    4. aripiprazole (Abilify)
    5. olanzapine (Zyprexa)

Objective: Identify the common adverse effects that are observed with the use of antipsychotic medications.
NCLEX item type: multiple response
Cognitive skill: application

17. The nurse discusses with the patient in the scenario who is taking an antipsychotic drug to report to his healthcare provider which of these serious adverse effects? *(Select all that apply.)* *(273)*
    1. Seizures
    2. Urinary retention
    3. Constipation
    4. Tardive dyskinesia
    5. Orthostatic hypotension

Copyright © 2023 by Elsevier, Inc. All rights reserved.

NCLEX item type: drop and drag

Cognitive skill: analyze cues

18. Patients taking antipsychotic medications may experience common adverse effects that the nurse can give instructions on.*(273)*

    Using an arrow, make a line from the common adverse effect to the instructions given by the nurse on how to manage the effects.

Common adverse effects	Instructions on how to manage adverse effects
Chronic fatigue	Suck on hard candy or ice chips
Drowsiness	Ensure safety with appropriate suggestions
Constipation	Do not work around machinery, or drive
Blurred vision	Eat high fiber diet, occasional laxative
Dry mouth	Take the dose of medication at bedtime

NCLEX item type: multiple choice

Cognitive skill: compare

19. A patient has been started on the atypical antipsychotic clozapine (Clozaril) for bipolar disorder. For the first 6 months of therapy, which lab result is most important for the nurse to monitor? *(273)*
    1. Red blood cell counts
    2. White blood cell counts
    3. Blood glucose
    4. Thyroid-stimulating hormone
    5. Prothrombin time

NCLEX item type: multiple choice

Cognitive skill: knowledge

20. Part of the teaching for the patient in the scenario, includes the nurse discussing dystonic reactions that may occur during which timeframe? *(Select all that apply.)* *(268)*
    1. Usually last for 1 week
    2. May not be responsive to treatment
    3. Occur most often in females
    4. Occur most often in the first 72 hours of therapy

Copyright © 2023 by Elsevier, Inc. All rights reserved.

Drugs Used for Seizure Disorders

chapter

18

Answer Key: Textbook page references are provided as a guide for answering these questions. A complete answer key is provided to your instructor.

MATCHING
Match the term on the right with the definition on the left.

Definition

1. _____ a rapidly recurring generalized seizure that does not allow the patient to regain normal function between seizures

2. _____ characterized by being awake and aware during a seizure

3. _____ recovery phase of flaccid paralysis and sleep

4. _____ bilaterally symmetric jerks alternating with the relaxation of the extremities

5. _____ a sudden loss of muscle tone, or drop attack

6. _____ a diagnosis applied to patients with chronic and recurrent seizures

7. _____ lightning-like repetitive contractions of the voluntary muscles of the face, trunk, and extremities

8. _____ a back-and-forth movement of the eyeballs on a horizontal plane

9. _____ intense muscular contractions; patients may fall, lose consciousness, and lie rigid

Term

a. epilepsy
b. nystagmus
c. postictal state
d. tonic phase
e. clonic phase
f. status epilepticus
g. atonic seizure
h. myoclonic seizure
i. focal seizures

REVIEW QUESTIONS

Scenario #1: A 32-year-old patient was admitted to the hospital following an episode of a generalized seizure witnessed by the family. The patient has been poorly controlled on their previous dosage of antiepileptic medications.

Objective: Identify the different types of seizure disorders.

NCLEX item type: multiple response
Cognitive skill: application

10. The nurse monitoring patients with known epilepsy reviewed the types of seizures. Seizures can be categorized by their presentation and is it not uncommon for patients to lose their balance and fall with no loss of consciousness. Which seizures does this describe **(277)** *(Select all that apply.)*
    1. Tonic-clonic
    2. Myoclonic
    3. Atonic
    4. Absence
    5. Focal

NCLEX item type: multiple choice
Cognitive skill: compare

11. When monitoring the patient in scenario #1 during a seizure, the nurse knows that generalized seizures such a tonic-clonic seizures are characterized as what? **(277)**
    1. Intense muscular contractions that cause a fall
    2. Bilateral jerks alternating with relaxation of the extremities
    3. A sudden loss of muscle tone, occurring in short attacks
    4. Lightning-like repetitive contractions of the muscles of the face

NCLEX item type: multiple choice
Cognitive skill: knowledge

12. The nurse discusses with a patient and their family that there is a type of seizure that is considered a medical emergency and prompt treatment is necessary to prevent nerve damage and death and explained it as which type? **(277)**
    1. Myoclonic seizures
    2. Tonic-clonic seizures
    3. Absence seizures
    4. Status epilepticus

Copyright © 2023 by Elsevier, Inc. All rights reserved.

NCLEX item type: recognize cues
Cognitive skill: grid/matrix

13. The nurse explains the difference between the types of seizures to the family of the patient in scenario #1 and identified that seizures are divided into classifications *(276-277)*
Indicate with an 'X' the classification of each type of seizure

	Focal (partial) seizures	Generalized seizures Convulsive	Generalized seizures Nonconvulsive
Absence			
Tonic-clonic			
Focal onset aware			
Myoclonic			
Focal impaired awareness			
Atonic			

Objective: Identify nursing interventions during the management of seizure activity.

NCLEX item type: multiple choice
Cognitive skill: take action

14. Which action does the nurse take when working with a patient experiencing a seizure? *(280)*
    1. Restrains the patient and places a tongue blade in the patient's mouth
    2. Medicates the patient immediately and observes for signs of recovery
    3. Asks the family to leave the room if present, and calmly waits outside the room for the seizure to stop
    4. Once the patient enters into the recovery phase, turns him or her slightly onto the side to allow secretions to drain from the mouth

NCLEX item type: multiple choice
Cognitive skill: interpret

15. The nurse is discussing the diagnosis of epilepsy to parents of a 5-year-old child who had been recently diagnosed with tonic-clonic seizures. Which statement by the parents indicates that the nurse needs to educate further? *(277)*
    1. "These seizures will be outgrown later in life."
    2. "Seizures are classified into focal onset, generalized onset and unknown onset."
    3. "*Epilepsy* is the general term meaning that the seizures are chronic."
    4. "The tonic-clonic seizures that were diagnosed have a recovery stage."

NCLEX item type: multiple response
Cognitive skill: application

16. The nurse needs to document what is happening to the patient in scenario #1 during a seizure and includes which information regarding the seizure? *(Select all that apply.) (279)*
    1. Duration of the seizure
    2. Progression of symptoms
    3. Onset or possible causal factor
    4. State of consciousness
    5. Which hemisphere of the brain is being affected

Objective: Discuss the desired therapeutic outcomes from antiepileptic agents used for seizure disorders.

NCLEX item type: multiple response
Cognitive skill: application

17. When administering antiepileptic agents to the patient in scenario #1, the nurse knows that the therapeutic outcomes include what? *(Select all that apply.) (281)*
    1. A reduced frequency of seizures
    2. A reduction in any injury from seizure activity
    3. Minimal adverse effects from therapy
    4. A reduction in tension and stress
    5. An alleviation of any seizure activity

NCLEX item type: multiple response
Cognitive skill: compare

18. The nurse reviews the drugs that are often used for the initial treatment of a newly diagnosed seizure disorder. Which medications are typical for this? *(Select all that apply.) (278)*
    1. lorazepam (Ativan)
    2. gabapentin (Neurontin)
    3. lamotrigine (Lamictal)
    4. topiramate (Topamax)
    5. levetiracetam (Keppra)

Scenario #2: A patient who has have a long history of epilepsy is following up on the change of medications that was ordered by their healthcare provider. The nurse is interviewing the patient and gathering important data regarding their seizure history and medications.

Objective: Identify the drug classes used to treat seizure disorders.

NCLEX item type: multiple response
Cognitive skill: application

19. The patient in scenario # 2 had been taking benzodiazepines for the treatment of their seizures because these medications are thought to have what effect? *(281)*
    1. Blocks the reuptake of norepinephrine
    2. Acts on voltage-gated potassium channels
    3. Blocks the voltage-gated calcium channels
    4. Enhance the effects of gamma-aminobutyric acid (GABA)

Copyright © 2023 by Elsevier, Inc. All rights reserved.

NCLEX item type: multiple choice
Cognitive skill: interpret

20. The nurse knows that succinimides are drugs that are used to decrease the frequency of seizures by which mechanism of action? *(285)*
    1. Enhancing the effects of GABA
    2. Blocking the reuptake of norepinephrine
    3. Blocking voltage-sensitive sodium
    4. Reducing the current in the T-type calcium channels

NCLEX item type: multiple choice
Cognitive skill: compare

21. The nurse reviewed the medication list of the patient in scenario #2 and recognized carbamazepine (Tegretol) as one the miscellaneous antiepileptic agent that works by which mechanism of action? *(286)*
    1. By blocking the voltage-gated calcium channels
    2. By blocking the reuptake of norepinephrine
    3. By enhancing the effectiveness of GABA
    4. By blocking the voltage-sensitive sodium channels

NCLEX item type: multiple choice
Cognitive skill: classify

22. The anticonvulsant lamotrigine, unrelated to other antiepileptic medications, is thought to act by blocking voltage-sensitive sodium and calcium channels, and is part of which class of drugs? *(288)*
    1. Hydantoins
    2. Phenyltriazine
    3. Succinimides
    4. Pyrrolidines

Objective: Describe the neurologic assessment performed on patients taking antiepileptic agents to monitor for common and serious adverse effects.

NCLEX item type: multiple choice
Cognitive skill: explain

23. The nurse is teaching the patient in scenario #1 about the use of phenytoin (Dilantin) for seizure control. What does the nurse tell the patient about taking oral contraceptives with this medication? *(285)*
    1. "You will not be able to become pregnant because of the phenytoin therapy."
    2. "There are no contraindications for using these two drugs together."
    3. "Dilantin therapy should be stopped if you experience spotting or bleeding."
    4. "An alternative form of birth control should be used when taking phenytoin with oral contraceptives."

NCLEX item type: multiple choice
Cognitive skill: explain

24. The patient in scenario # 1 is also diabetic and taking hydantoins. The nurse will need to educate the patient on the risk of which complication? *(284)*
    1. Developing oral thrush
    2. Decreased effectiveness of hydantoin
    3. Hyperglycemia with hydantoin therapy
    4. Increased frequency of hypoglycemia

NCLEX item type: multiple choice
Cognitive skill: comprehension

25. When patients are on antacids and hydantoins, they should be told that the antacid will have what effect? *(285)*
    1. Decrease the therapeutic effect of phenytoin
    2. Increase the therapeutic effect of phenytoin
    3. Increase the level of hydantoin in the blood, causing toxicity
    4. Decrease the therapeutic effects of the antacid

NCLEX item type: multiple response
Cognitive skill: application

26. The nurse assessing the patient in scenario #2 who is starting on topiramate (Topamax) knows to monitor for which common adverse effects? *(Select all that apply.)* *(294)*
    1. Sedation
    2. Dizziness
    3. Drowsiness
    4. Constipation
    5. Increased sweating

NCLEX item type: multiple choice
Cognitive skill: knowledge

27. When the patient is started on an antiepileptic drug, the nurse needs to closely monitor for which adverse effect that may occur as early as 1 week or as late as several months? *(279)*
    1. Suicidal ideation
    2. Increased appetite along with increased energy
    3. Increase in muscle soreness and extreme need for sleep
    4. Halitosis, requiring increase frequency of oral hygiene

Copyright © 2023 by Elsevier, Inc. All rights reserved.

Drugs Used for Pain Management

Answer Key: Textbook page references are provided as a guide for answering these questions. A complete answer key is provided to your instructor.

MATCHING
Match the definition on the right with the term on the left.

Term

1. _____ pain experience
2. _____ neuropathic pain
3. _____ pain perception
4. _____ idiopathic pain
5. _____ pain threshold
6. _____ analgesics
7. _____ opiate agonists
8. _____ pain tolerance
9. _____ opiate antagonists

Definition

a. pain that results from injury to the peripheral or central nervous system
b. the individual's ability to endure pain
c. a group of naturally occurring and synthetic substances that relieve severe pain without loss of consciousness
d. an unpleasant sensation that is highly subjective and influenced by sensory, emotional, and cultural factors
e. nonspecific pain of unknown origin
f. the point at which an individual first acknowledges or interprets a sensation of pain
g. drugs that have no other known effect than reversal of the CNS depressant effects of opiate agonists
h. an individual's awareness of the feeling or sensation of pain
i. drugs that relieve pain without producing loss of consciousness

REVIEW QUESTIONS

Scenario #1: A patient recovering from a recent fall that resulted in broken vertebrae and the need for a 'turtle shell' for back support was talking with a nurse about pain control.

Objective: Describe the pain assessment used for patients receiving opiate agonists.

NCLEX item type: multiple choice
Cognitive skill: interpret

10. The nurse taking care of the patient in scenario #1 is discussing various pain management options with the patient and realizes more education is needed when the patient makes which statement? *(304,308)*
    1. "I am pretty sure this tablet will not take away my pain, I know I need IV medications."
    2. "One of the goals I have for pain relief is to be able to sleep at least 6 hours without waking up."
    3. "I know I need to eat a well-balanced diet and drink plenty of water while taking codeine."
    4. "I understand I can use other measures to relieve pain in addition to taking this codeine, like a heating pad."

NCLEX item type: multiple response
Cognitive skill: application

11. For patients taking opiate agonists, the nurse needs to monitor the patient for signs of which adverse effects? *(Select all that apply.)* *(311,315)*
    1. Diarrhea
    2. Hyperglycemia
    3. Urinary retention
    4. Respiratory depression
    5. Confusion or disorientation

NCLEX item type: multiple response
Cognitive skill: analyze

12. When determining if the patient in scenario #1 has pain, the nurse needs to assess which components of the pain assessment? *(Select all that apply.)* *(305,307)*
    1. The location of pain
    2. The rating on a pain scale
    3. The duration of pain
    4. The quality of pain
    5. The last time no pain was felt

Copyright © 2023 by Elsevier, Inc. All rights reserved.

Objective: Differentiate among the properties of opiate agonists, opiate partial agonists, and opiate antagonists.

NCLEX item type: multiple choice
Cognitive skill: compare

13. The nurse understands that opiate agonists interact with receptors to stimulate a response of pain relief, whereas partial agonists may do what? *(316)*
    1. Block any response
    2. Induce a stupor or sleep
    3. Stimulate a response, but may inhibit other responses
    4. Induce withdrawal symptoms if any opiate agonist has been given

NCLEX item type: multiple choice
Cognitive skill: compare

14. The nurse reviews the drug naloxone an opiate antagonists for its mechanism of action. What does the nurse find as the correct action? *(318)*
    1. Opiate antagonists block the effects of any euphoric high
    2. Opiate antagonists stimulate a response of pain relief
    3. Opiate antagonists reverse the depressant effects of any opiate agonist
    4. Opiate antagonists stimulate a response, but may inhibit other responses

NCLEX item type: multiple choice
Cognitive skill: knowledge

15. The nurse knows which statement is true about the use of the transdermal opioid analgesic fentanyl (Duragesic)? *(313)*
    1. Fentanyl is only used for acute pain.
    2. Fentanyl patches provide relief for up to 72 hours.
    3. No other analgesics may be used concurrently with fentanyl.
    4. Approximately 2 hours are required for the initial patch of medication to reach a steady blood level.

Objective: Discuss the common adverse effects of opiate agonists.

NCLEX item type: extended multiple response
Cognitive skill: recognize cues

16. The patient in scenario #1 is receiving opiate agonists for pain control. Which common adverse effect does the nurse learn how to manage? *(Select all that apply.) (311,315)*
    1. Nausea
    2. Lightheadedness
    3. Respiratory rate of 7
    4. Excessive use
    5. Constipation
    6. Sweating
    7. Urinary retention
    8. Orthostatic hypotension

NCLEX item type: multiple choice
Cognitive skill: relate

17. The nurse educated the patient taking an opioid regarding a common adverse effect can usually be treated by diet and stool softeners. Which complication was the nurse referring to? *(315)*
    1. Constipation
    2. Urinary retention
    3. Respiratory depression
    4. Orthostatic hypotension

NCLEX item type: multiple choice
Cognitive skill: explain

18. What should the nurse instruct patients who report lightheadedness and dizziness after the first dose of hydromorphone (Dilaudid) to do? *(311)*
    1. Remain lying down.
    2. Increase the amount of whole-grain products in their diet.
    3. Report this effect to the healthcare provider for further evaluation.
    4. Sit up quickly and stand after 30 seconds of sitting to relieve symptoms.

NCLEX item type: multiple response
Cognitive skill: application

19. If an opiate partial agonist (nalbuphine) is administered to a patient who is addicted to the opiate agonist (oxycodone), what must the nurse assess for? *(316)*
    1. Constipation
    2. Hypotension
    3. Elevated WBCs
    4. Withdrawal symptoms

NCLEX item type: multiple choice
Cognitive skill: contrast

20. The nurse reviewed the drugs that are antidotes for opiate agonists and opiate partial agonists and removed which two drugs to use as antidotes? *(318)*
    1. Naloxone (Narcan) and pentazocine
    2. Naltrexone (ReVia) and nalbuphine
    3. Naloxone (Narcan) and naltrexone (ReVia)
    4. Naltrexone (ReVia) and butorphanol

NCLEX item type: multiple choice
Cognitive skill: interpret

21. The patient in scenario #1 asks the nurse about the drug pentazocine/naloxone a opiate partial agonists how effective it is in relieving pain. Which response by the nurse needs to be corrected? *(316)*
    1. "The drug pentazocine/naloxone works just a well as the opiate agonists for pain relief."
    2. "We will sometimes give drugs such as pentazocine/naloxone to people who find that opiate agonists are no longer effective."
    3. "The drugs such as pentazocine/naloxone which are opiate partial agonists can be used for patients after surgery in conjunction with opiate agonists."
    4. "The drug pentazocine/naloxone will have effective pain relief in cases where patients are physically dependent on opioids."

Copyright © 2023 by Elsevier, Inc. All rights reserved.

Objective: Identify opiate antagonists and expected therapeutic outcomes to monitor.

NCLEX item type: multiple choice

Cognitive skill: knowledge

22. Emergency service personnel across the nation now carry the opiate antagonist naloxone (Narcan) for cases of what? *(318)*
    1. Acute hemorrhage after motor vehicle accidents
    2. Food poisoning from poor food handling
    3. Acute anaphylaxis by bee stings
    4. Respiratory depression from overdoses of opiates

NCLEX item type: extended multiple response

Cognitive skill: analysis cues

23. The nurse reviews the adverse effect of naloxone (Narcan). Which effects usually occur in the first few days of treatment and dissipates rapidly? *(Select all that apply.)* *(318)*
    1. Inability to concentrate
    2. Respiratory depression
    3. Irritability
    4. Sleepiness
    5. Anorexia
    6. Constipation
    7. Vomiting
    8. Hypertension

NCLEX item type: cloze

Cognitive skill: evaluate

24. **Choose the most likely options for the information missing from the statements below by selecting from the list of options provided.**

The nurse reviewed the drugs in the class of

_____1_____ and recognized the drug

_____2_____ is the one that can be given orally for patients with respiratory depression secondary to opiate overdose. *(318)*

Option 1	Option 2
opiates	naproxen
opiate agonists	naloxone
opiate antagonists	nabumetone
opiate partial agonists	naltrexone

Scenario #2: A patient with a headache, muscle aches and a recent sinus infection come to the Urgent Care clinic to seek the advice of the nurse regarding what would be most effective medications to relieve their symptoms.

Objective: Describe the three pharmacologic effects of salicylates.

NCLEX item type: multiple choice

Cognitive skill: compare

25. The nurse discussed with the patient in scenario #2 the effects aspirin has which make it a versatile medication. Which pharmacologic properties does the nurse describe? *(321)*
    1. Antiepileptic, antiplatelet, and antiinflammatory
    2. Analgesic, antiplatelet, and antacid
    3. Analgesic, antipyretic, and antiinflammatory
    4. Antiinflammatory, antipyretic, and antacid

NCLEX item type: multiple response

Cognitive skill: application

26. The nurse describes examples of conditions that aspirin or any salicylate can be used for with the patient in scenario #2. Which conditions does the nurse describe? *(Select all that apply.)* *(321)*
    1. "Salicylates are used to help reduce fever from infections, such as a sinus infection."
    2. "For patients who have inflammation from rheumatoid arthritis, salicylates are very useful."
    3. "We can use salicylates to prevent the symptoms of withdrawal from opiates."
    4. Reduce the risk of recurrent TIA or stroke
    5. Reduce the risk of myocardial infarction

NCLEX item type: multiple response

Cognitive skill: evaluate

27. The nurse knows that salicylates work by inhibiting prostaglandins. What assessments does the nurse perform prior to administration of aspirin or aspirin like products? *(Select all that apply.)* *(321-322)*
    1. Baseline neurologic assessment
    2. Determine the degree of mobility
    3. Perform a pain assessment
    4. Determine concurrent use of anticoagulant agents
    5. Auscultate heart and lung sounds

Copyright © 2023 by Elsevier, Inc. All rights reserved.

Objective: Compare the common and serious adverse effects and drug interactions associated with salicylates.

NCLEX item type: multiple choice
Cognitive skill: relate

28. A patient has been taking an oral hypoglycemic agent and is being started on salicylate therapy for pain management. Which statement does the nurse use to explain what will happen when these two types of drugs are taken together? *(322)*
    1. "You will need to switch to subcutaneous insulin therapy for the duration of the salicylate therapy."
    2. "When you take oral hypoglycemic agents they will potentiate the effect of the salicylates and increase the chance of salicylate toxicity."
    3. "If you are on an oral hypoglycemic agent your dose will be doubled while you take the salicylate therapy."
    4. "As I understand it salicylates may enhance the hypoglycemic effects of oral hypoglycemic agents; therefore, the dose may need to be reduced."

NCLEX item type: multiple choice
Cognitive skill: explain

29. The parents of a 5-year-old child asked the nurse why salicylates should not be used for children. Which statement by the nurse is accurate? *(321)*
    1. "Children should not receive salicylates because there is an increased chance of overdosing them."
    2. "Aspirin and aspirin like medications should not be given to children because of the associated risk of Reye's syndrome."
    3. "Children are susceptible to developing a toxic response from salicylates."
    4. "When children are given salicylates they have an increased risk for developing respiratory depression."

NCLEX item type: multiple response
Cognitive skill: application

30. The nurse is aware that salicylates should not be given to patients with which conditions? *(Select all that apply.)* *(322)*
    1. Peptic ulcers
    2. Glaucoma
    3. Liver disease
    4. Coagulation disorders
    5. Previous myocardial infarctions

NCLEX item type: multiple choice
Cognitive skill: compare

31. When comparing the therapeutic effects of NSAIDs to acetaminophen (Tylenol), the nurse knows that both are very good antipyretic and analgesic agents; however what is the difference? *(320)*
    1. Acetaminophen has antiplatelet effects.
    2. NSAIDs have antiplatelet effects.
    3. Acetaminophen has no antiinflammatory effect.
    4. NSAIDs have no effect on prostaglandins.

NCLEX item type: multiple choice
Cognitive skill: comprehension

32. The nurse knows the primary therapeutic outcomes expected from acetaminophen (Tylenol) include what affect? *(320)*
    1. Reduction of inflammation and pain
    2. Reduction of pain and fever
    3. Relief of pain and heartburn
    4. Improvement of circulation and nasal congestion

NCLEX item type: multiple choice
Cognitive skill: knowledge

33. The nurse is explaining to the patient in scenario #2 that the active ingredients in Anacin include what drugs? *(326)*
    1. Aspirin and caffeine
    2. Aspirin and hydrocodone
    3. Acetaminophen and aspirin
    4. Acetaminophen and caffeine

Copyright © 2023 by Elsevier, Inc. All rights reserved.

Introduction to Cardiovascular Disease and Metabolic Syndrome

chapter
20

Answer Key: Textbook page references are provided as a guide for answering these questions. A complete answer key is provided to your instructor.

MATCHING
Match the term on the right with the definition on the left.

Definitions

1. _____ abnormalities in the electrical conduction pathways of the heart

2. _____ a narrowing or obstruction of the arteries of the heart

3. _____ an obstruction or rupture of blood vessels in the brain

4. _____ a collective term used to refer to disorders of the circulatory system

5. _____ involves disorders of the blood vessels of the arms and legs

6. _____ an increase in the pressure with which blood circulates through the arteries

7. _____ weight in proportion to height

Terms

a. hypertension
b. dysrhythmias
c. coronary artery disease
d. peripheral vascular disease
e. stroke
f. body mass index (BMI)
g. cardiovascular disease

REVIEW QUESTIONS

Scenario #1: A 42-year-old male patient discusses with the nurse the need for exercising, as he had previously indicated that he rarely exercises. The nurse asked questions designed to get him to think about why he does not exercise and what some of his beliefs are about this, as he is obese and just diagnosed with hypertension.

Objective: Identify the major risk factors for the development of metabolic syndrome.
NCLEX item type: multiple response
Cognitive skill: application

8. The nurse will explain to the patient in scenario #1 the risk factors that he needs to consider that may lead to the development of metabolic syndrome, which include what factors? *(Select all that apply.)* **(330)**
   1. Obesity
   2. Diabetes
   3. Hypertension
   4. Active lifestyle
   5. Stressful occupation

NCLEX item type: multiple response
Cognitive skill: compare

9. The nurse explained to the patient in scenario #1 the cardiovascular disorders which are attributed to the narrowing or obstruction of the arteries of the heart that include which conditions? *(Select all that apply.)* **(330)**
   1. Stroke
   2. Hypertension
   3. Angina pectoris
   4. Myocardial infarction
   5. Peripheral vascular disease

NCLEX item type: multiple response
Cognitive skill: application

10. In addition to type 2 diabetes and heart disease, the nurse discusses with the patient in the scenario that other consequences are associated with metabolic syndrome. Which medical conditions will the nurse identify? *(Select all that apply.)* **(331)**
    1. Renal disease
    2. Liver disease
    3. Obstructive sleep apnea
    4. Cognitive decline in older adults
    5. Polycystic ovary syndrome

Copyright © 2023 by Elsevier, Inc. All rights reserved.

NCLEX item type: multiple response
Cognitive skill: illustrate

11. After teaching the patient about peripheral vascular disease involving disorders of the blood vessels of the arms and legs the nurse asks the patient to name some. Which medical conditions did the patient identify? *(Select all that apply.)* *(330)*
    1. Stroke
    2. Diabetes
    3. Myocardial infarction
    4. Obstructive arterial disease
    5. Deep vein thrombosis

Objective: Discuss the importance of lifestyle modification in the management of metabolic syndrome.

NCLEX item type: drag and drop
Cognitive skill: analyze cues

12. The nurse encourages the patient in scenario #1 regarding lifestyle modifications that can help control the development of metabolic syndrome and teach health promotion. *(332)*

Indicate with an 'X' which suggestion would be an appropriate lifestyle modification and which would have no apparent benefit.

	Appropriate lifestyle modification	No apparent benefit
Smoking cessation		
Sedentary activity		
Excessive alcohol		
Stress reduction		
Weight reduction		
Healthy diet		
Increased caloric intake		

NCLEX item type: multiple response
Cognitive skill: application

13. When teaching the patient in scenario #1 about metabolic syndrome, the nurse discusses ways to promote weight loss and increase physical activity. Which statements by the nurse are accurate methods to encourage the patient to try? *(Select all that apply.)* *(332,334)*
    1. "If you adopt the DASH diet it has been effective in helping people to lose weight."
    2. "One suggestion would be to reduce the number of calories that you eat at each meal."
    3. "If you exercise at the same time of day consistently, you should be able to lose weight."
    4. "It is recommended to get 60 minutes of moderate-intensity physical activity twice a week."
    5. "When determining what to eat, the fat in your diet should be unsaturated, and simple sugars should be reduced to a minimum."

NCLEX item type: multiple response
Cognitive skill: interpret

14. The patient asks the nurse about examples of some of the characteristics of a sedentary lifestyle that contribute to obesity and the development of metabolic syndrome. Which response should the nurse include in the discussion? *(Select all that apply.)* *(332)*
    1. Work-related stress
    2. Labor-saving devices
    3. Remote control devices
    4. Genetic predisposition
    5. Entertainment through television and computers

Scenario #2: An obese patient being seen in the clinic for management of diabetes and hypertension mentions to the nurse that they are having trouble keeping the blood sugar under 150.

Objective: Explain the treatment goals for type 2 diabetes management, lipid management, and hypertension management.

NCLEX item type: multiple response
Cognitive skill: analyze

15. The nurse reviewed the overall treatment goals with the patient in scenario #2 for metabolic syndrome and knows they include which parameters? *(Select all that apply.)* *(335)*
    1. LDL of < 100 mg/dL
    2. Hemoglobin A1C levels < 7%
    3. Triglyceride levels of < 150 mg/dL
    4. Fasting blood sugar of < 120 mg/dL
    5. Blood pressure of < 130/80 mm Hg

NCLEX item type: multiple choice
Cognitive skill: explain

16. When teaching the patient in scenario #2 with metabolic syndrome about the importance of weight loss and a healthy diet, the nurse includes which statement? *(332)*
    1. "Olive oil is an example of the type of 'good' fat you may eat."
    2. "Most of the dietary fat you consume should be saturated."
    3. "You must limit the amount of protein you eat to 2 ounces once a day."
    4. "Restrict the total amount of fat you consume each day to approximately 45% of your total calories."

NCLEX item type: multiple choice
Cognitive skill: interpret

17. The nurse is reviewing the lab values that indicate that the general treatment goals for patients with metabolic syndrome are being met. Which lab value will the nurse expect to see? *(335)*
    1. Hemoglobin A1C of 8.5%
    2. Postprandial plasma glucose of 190 mg/dL
    3. Hemoglobin A1C of 5%
    4. Fasting plasma glucose of 138 mg/dL

Copyright © 2023 by Elsevier, Inc. All rights reserved.

Objective: Discuss the drug management of the underlying diseases used by patients with metabolic syndrome.

NCLEX item type: multiple response
Cognitive skill: application

18. The nurse reviews the treatment for hypertension when changes in diet and exercise do not produce acceptable reduction in blood pressure include which drug class? *(Select all that apply.)* **(335)**
    1. Analgesics
    2. Thiazide diuretics
    3. Calcium channel blockers
    4. Alpha-glucosidase inhibitors
    5. Angiotensin-converting enzyme inhibitors

NCLEX item type: multiple choice
Cognitive skill: classify

19. The nurse reviews the treatment for dyslipidemia is generally to lower the triglycerides and LDL cholesterol and raise the HDL cholesterol and includes which drug class? **(335)**
    1. Statins
    2. Thiazide diuretics
    3. Calcium channel blockers
    4. Alpha-glucosidase inhibitors

NCLEX item type: multiple choice
Cognitive skill: compare

20. The nurse knows that the drug classes used to treat type 2 diabetes mellitus associated with metabolic syndrome will stimulate the beta cells of the pancreas to release more insulin and are known as what? **(335)**
    1. Sulfonylureas and meglitinides
    2. Meglitinides and thiazolidinediones
    3. Thiazolidinediones and alpha-glucosidase inhibitors
    4. Sulfonylureas and thiazolidinediones

Copyright © 2023 by Elsevier, Inc. All rights reserved.

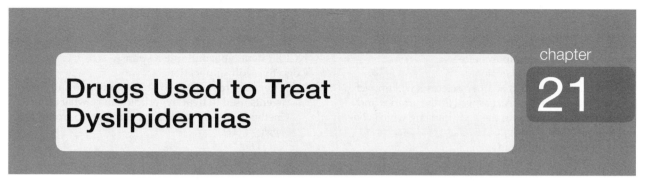

Drugs Used to Treat Dyslipidemias

chapter

21

Answer Key: Textbook page references are provided as a guide for answering these questions. A complete answer key is provided to your instructor.

MATCHING

Match the term on the right with the definition on the left.

Definition

1. _____ substance essential for synthesizing steroids and bile acids

2. _____ characterized by the accumulation of fatty deposits on the inner walls of blood vessels

3. _____ 90% triglycerides and 5% cholesterol

4. _____ lipids bound to circulating proteins

5. _____ a broad term used to classify patients with high levels of blood fats

6. _____ a precursor to cholesterol

Term

a. hyperlipidemia
b. atherosclerosis
c. triglycerides
d. chylomicrons
e. cholesterol
f. lipoproteins

REVIEW QUESTIONS

Scenario #1: An obese 58-year-old female patient with hypertension and diabetes was told during a routine checkup that she had elevated levels of cholesterol and needed to be started on antilipid therapy along with diet modification.

Objective: Describe atherosclerosis and identify the five major types of lipoproteins.
NCLEX item type: Extended multiple response
Cognitive skill: recognize cues

7. The nurse recognizes that the risk factors for developing atherosclerosis which are treatable, include which factors? (*Select all that apply.*) *(338)*
   1. Daily exercise
   2. Sedentary lifestyle
   3. Cigarette smoking
   4. Increased vitamin intake
   5. Poor eating habits
   6. Hypertension
   7. Type 2 diabetes
   8. Hypothyroidism

NCLEX item type: multiple response
Cognitive skill: application

8. The nurse discusses with the patient in scenario #1 that atherosclerosis is characterized by the accumulation of fatty deposits on the inner walls of arteries and arterioles throughout the body that reduce the blood supply to vital organs which can result in which conditions? (*Select all that apply.*) *(338)*
   1. Myocardial infarction
   2. Type 2 diabetes
   3. Angina pectoris
   4. Cardiac dysrhythmias
   5. Peripheral vascular disease

NCLEX item type: multiple choice
Cognitive skill: knowledge

9. The nurse reviews lipoproteins while educating the patient in scenario #1 and explains that there is one type that is referred to as the "good" lipoprotein because high levels indicate that cholesterol is being removed from vascular tissue. Which lipoprotein is the nurse describing? *(339)*
   1. IDL
   2. VLDL
   3. LDL
   4. HDL

Copyright © 2023 by Elsevier, Inc. All rights reserved.

NCLEX item type: multiple choice
Cognitive skill: comprehension

10. The nurse expects that atherosclerosis will impact the arteries of the heart as well as the arteries and arterioles throughout the body, causing which condition? *(338)*
    1. Urinary retention
    2. Erosive esophagitis
    3. Peripheral vascular disease
    4. Increased cerebral profusion

NCLEX item type: multiple choice
Cognitive skill: classify

11. The nurse discusses with the patient in scenario #1 that lipoproteins are subdivided into five categories based on composition: chylomicrons, very low-density lipoproteins (VLDLs), intermediate-density lipoproteins (IDLs), low-density lipoproteins (LDLs), and high-density lipoproteins (HDLs). The five types differ in relative concentrations of what substances? *(339)*
    1. Cholesterol, triglycerides, and steroids
    2. Triglycerides, proteins, and amino acids
    3. Cholesterol, protein, and carbohydrates
    4. Triglycerides, cholesterol, and proteins

NCLEX item type: multiple choice
Cognitive skill: knowledge

12. The nurse reviews with the patient in scenario #1 why low levels of HDLs are considered a positive risk factor for the development of which condition? *(339)*
    1. Diabetes
    2. Bleeding disorders
    3. Coronary artery disease
    4. Elevated C-reactive protein levels

Objective: Describe the primary approaches to treat lipid disorders.

NCLEX item type: multiple choice
Cognitive skill: illustrate

13. The patient in scenario #1 came back to the clinic for a checkup after starting atorvastatin (Lipitor) and asked the nurse how the drug works. Which statement by the nurse would be appropriate? *(342)*
    1. "The statins interfere with the absorption of cholesterol from the diet."
    2. "The statins inhibit an enzyme in the pathway to making cholesterol in the liver."
    3. "The statins work best when taken with another antilipid agent to lower your cholesterol level."
    4. "The exact action of statins is unknown, but they are effective agents in reducing cholesterol."

NCLEX item type: multiple response
Cognitive skill: application

14. The nurse remembers that in addition to antilipid agents used to treat hyperlipidemias, what other methods are employed for treatment? *(Select all that apply.)* *(342)*
    1. Diet
    2. Exercise
    3. Weight reduction
    4. Controlling blood pressure
    5. Regular dental checkups

NCLEX item type: cloze
Cognitive skill: recognize cues

15. **Choose the most likely options for the information missing from the statements below by selecting from the list of options provided.**

The nurse recognized the antilipid agent _____1_____ that is used in conjunction with _____2_____ to reduce elevated cholesterol concentration blocking the absorption of cholesterol by the small intestine. *(346)*

Option 1	Option 2
Omega-3 fatty acids (Lovaza)	Bile acid-binding resins
Simvastatin (Zocor)	Dietary therapy
Cholestyramine (Questran)	Physical therapy
Ezetimibe (Zetia)	Daily laxative

Scenario #2: A patient returned to the clinic for a routine checkup to follow up on how well they have been doing after starting on antilipemic agents to control their dyslipidemia.

Objective: Determine which antilipemic medications are used for cholesterol control and which can be used for triglyceride control.

NCLEX item type: multiple response
Cognitive skill: application

16. When teaching a patient about niacin therapy, the nurse tells the patient to report which adverse effects to the primary healthcare provider? *(Select all that apply.)* *(349)*
    1. Flushing
    2. Jaundice
    3. Muscle aches
    4. Headaches
    5. Abdominal discomfort

Copyright © 2023 by Elsevier, Inc. All rights reserved.

NCLEX item type: multiple response
Cognitive skill: relate

17. The nurse explains to the patient in scenario #1 that the statin drugs are the most potent antilipid agents available with which added benefits that result in decreased heart attacks and stroke? *(Select all that apply.)* **(343)**
    1. Decreased amounts of HDL
    2. Decreased inflammation
    3. Decreased platelet aggregation
    4. Decreased thrombin formation
    5. Decreased plasma viscosity

NCLEX item type: multiple choice
Cognitive skill: knowledge

18. The nurse knows that there are antilipid agents used to reduce triglyceride levels for patients who have hypertriglyceridemia. Which drug class is considered the most effective triglyceride-lowering agents? **(350)**
    1. Niacin
    2. Statins
    3. Fibric acids
    4. Bile acid–binding resins

Objective: Differentiate between how statins work to control lipid levels and how the bile acid resins work to control lipid levels.

NCLEX item type: multiple choice
Cognitive skill: relate

19. The nurse instructing the patient in scenario #1 taking a HMG-CoA reductase inhibitor for the treatment of hyperlipidemia, reminded her to do what? **(344-345)**
    1. Avoid drinking grapefruit juice.
    2. Have liver function tests monitored every 2 months.
    3. Expect muscle weakness as a common adverse effect.
    4. Take the medication on an empty stomach to increase absorption.

NCLEX item type: multiple response
Cognitive skill: explain

20. The patient in scenario #2 who has been taking a bile acid–binding resin for the treatment of dyslipidemia tells the nurse that ever since they began taking the medication, they have been experiencing bloating and fullness. What does the nurse instruct the patient to do? *(Select all that apply.)* **(345)**
    1. Limit fluid intake.
    2. Start the medication with a low dose.
    3. Swallow the medication without gulping air.
    4. Maintain adequate fiber in the diet.
    5. Mix the medication with a carbonated beverage.

Copyright © 2023 by Elsevier, Inc. All rights reserved.

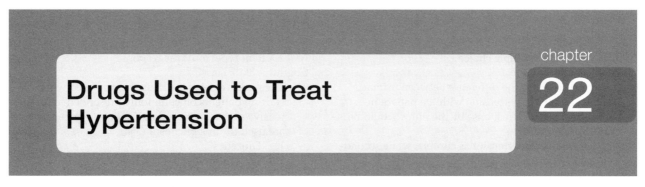

Drugs Used to Treat Hypertension

chapter 22

Answer Key: Textbook page references are provided as a guide for answering these questions. A complete answer key is provided to your instructor.

MATCHING

Match the term on the right with the definition on the left.

Definition

1. _____ a disease characterized by an elevation of the blood pressure
2. _____ the most common form of hypertension
3. _____ drugs that bind to angiotensin II receptor sites
4. _____ the difference between the systolic and diastolic pressure
5. _____ drugs that cause volume depletion, sodium excretion, and vasodilation of peripheral arterioles
6. _____ the pressure in the blood vessels when the heart muscle relaxes between contractions
7. _____ drugs that cause arteriolar smooth muscle relaxation
8. _____ high blood pressure that occurs after the development of another disorder
9. _____ drugs that inhibit angiotensin I converting enzyme
10. _____ drugs that inhibit cardiac response to sympathetic nerve stimulation by blocking beta receptors
11. _____ the pressure with which the blood is pumped from the heart
12. _____ drugs that inhibit the movement of calcium ions across a cell membrane
13. _____ this accounts for 90% of all clinical cases of high blood pressure, cause unknown
14. _____ this is determined by the stroke volume, heart rate, and venous capacitance
15. _____ the average pressure throughout each cycle of the heartbeat

Term

a. secondary hypertension
b. pulse pressure
c. systolic blood pressure
d. mean arterial pressure
e. diastolic blood pressure
f. hypertension
g. beta-adrenergic blockers
h. cardiac output
i. primary hypertension
j. systolic hypertension
k. diuretic
l. ACE inhibitors
m. angiotensin II receptor blockers
n. calcium channel blockers
o. direct vasodilators

REVIEW QUESTIONS

Scenario #1: A 42-year-old man came into the clinic complaining of frequent headaches and was diagnosed with stage 1 hypertension. He was referred to the education specialist for further instructions on lifestyle modification and initiation of drug therapy.

Objective: Differentiate between primary and secondary hypertension.

NCLEX item type: multiple choice
Cognitive skill: classify

16. A patient in the scenario #1 has a blood pressure reading of 138/85 mm Hg. The nurse identifies this patient as having which classification of hypertension? *(355)*
    1. Normal
    2. Stage 1
    3. Stage 2
    4. Elevated

Copyright © 2023 by Elsevier, Inc. All rights reserved.

NCLEX item type: multiple choice
Cognitive skill: compare
17. A nurse discusses the difference between primary and secondary hypertension with the patient in scenario #1. Which response by the nurse would be appropriate? *(354)*
    1. "Primary hypertension is curable, while secondary hypertension is only controllable."
    2. "There is no difference between primary and secondary hypertension; both of them can be cured."
    3. "Primary hypertension occurs during adolescence, while secondary hypertension happens to people after they reach adulthood."
    4. "Primary hypertension occurs about 90% of the time and has no known cause, while secondary hypertension occurs after the development of another disorder."

NCLEX item type: multiple choice
Cognitive skill: explain
18. The nurse explains to the patient in scenario #1 that systolic blood pressure is the pressure exerted by the heart as blood is pumped out. How will the nurse explain diastolic blood pressure? *(353)*
    1. "This is the pressure throughout each cycle of the heartbeat."
    2. "This pressure occurs when the blood is pumped from the right ventricle through the pulmonary artery."
    3. "This is the pressure that is calculated by adding one-third of the pulse pressure to the arterial pressure."
    4. "This refers to when the heart muscle relaxes between contractions."

NCLEX item type: multiple response
Cognitive skill: application
19. The nurse understands there are other conditions that are identifiable as causes of hypertension. Which conditions are possible? *(Select all that apply.)* *(354)*
    1. Sleep apnea
    2. Chronic kidney disease
    3. Primary aldosteronism
    4. Marfan's syndrome
    5. Thyroid disease

Objective: Summarize nursing assessments and interventions used for the treatment of hypertension.
NCLEX item type: multiple response
Cognitive skill: illustrate
20. What will the nurse do to measure a patient's blood pressure? *(Select all that apply.)* *(354)*
    1. Use an appropriately sized cuff.
    2. Verify reading in the opposite arm.
    3. Support the arm at the same level as the heart.
    4. Sit the patient in a chair with feet dangling off the floor.
    5. Inflate the cuff 50 mm Hg above the point at which the radial pulse disappears.

NCLEX item type: multiple response
Cognitive skill: classify
21. The nurse reviews the drug therapy used when starting patients on commonly prescribed antihypertensive agents. Which classification of medications are used for this purpose? *(356)*
    1. Diuretics
    2. ACE inhibitors
    3. Alpha-1 adrenergic blocking agents
    4. Angiotensin II receptor blockers
    5. Calcium channel blockers

NCLEX item type: multiple response
Cognitive skill: application
22. The nurse will assess those patients who are diagnosed with hypertension, for further evaluation of what? *(Select all that apply.)* ()
    1. Any history of risk factors, such a family history
    2. Any current medications to determine drug-drug interaction potential
    3. Determine patient's type of lifestyle; stress level, exercise routine, etc.
    4. Current understanding of the drugs used for hypertension
    5. Elevated serum lipid levels and renal function studies

NCLEX item type: multiple response
Cognitive skill: ordering
23. The nurse reviews the renin angiotensin aldosterone system (RAAS) to gain a better understanding of the various types of antihypertensive agents and what effect they have on this system. List in order the correct sequence of reactions that occur in the RAAS. *(364)*
    1. _____ angiotensin I is converted by angiotensin I-converting enzyme to angiotensin II
    2. _____ aldosterone causes sodium retention
    3. _____ angiotensinogen is converted by renin to form angiotensin I
    4. _____ angiotensin II promotes aldosterone secretion
    5. _____ renin is released by the kidneys NCLEX item type: multiple response

Cognitive skill: application
24. The nurse educates the patient in scenario #1 regarding what to do when taking hypertension medication. Which instructions will be included in the teaching? *(Select all that apply.)* *(362)*
    1. "You will need to know the correct dose to take for your medication."
    2. "It is important to know when you are to take these drugs so you can remember the time to take them and how often."
    3. "We will go over the common adverse effects to watch for when taking these medications."
    4. "It is important for you to check your temperature every day."
    5. "I will teach you when you should perform toe wiggles and rising up on your toes."

Copyright © 2023 by Elsevier, Inc. All rights reserved.

Scenario #2: A patient evaluated in the clinic for ongoing hypertension management also has the diagnosis of diabetes and being overweight. The patient mentioned the stress of a job was causing fatigue and sleep was a problem.

Objective: Identify recommended lifestyle modifications after a diagnosis of hypertension.
NCLEX item type: cloze
Cognitive skill: recognize cues
25. **Choose the most likely options for the information missing from the statements below by selecting from the list of options provided.**
The nurse explains to the patient in scenario #2 that _____1_____ and _____1_____ may be the result of uncontrolled hypertension, and it is important to treat hypertension with _____2_____ and _____2_____.*(354)*

Option 1	Option 2
Bladder cancer	Lifestyle modifications
Heart failure	Blood pressure monitoring
Hyperthyroidism	Antihypertensive medications
Stroke	Determining peripheral pulses

NCLEX item type: multiple response
Cognitive skill: evaluate cues
26. The nurse discusses the modifications that are recommended for the patient in scenario #2. Which statements by the nurse are appropriate? *(Select all that apply.)* *(355)*
    1. Weight reduction
    2. Using the DASH diet
    3. Stress management training
    4. Maintaining usual sodium intake
    5. Increase physical activity to moderate exercise
NCLEX item type: multiple response
Cognitive skill: application
27. The nurse discusses lifestyle modifications for the patient in scenario #2 regarding the treatment of hypertension. Which suggestions are appropriate for the nurse to recommend? *(Select all that apply.)* *(356)*
    1. Eating more fruits and vegetables
    2. Consuming more dairy products per day
    3. Reducing the amount of dietary sodium intake
    4. Limiting consumption of alcohol to no more than two drinks per day
    5. Increasing physical activity to 40 minutes, three or four times per week

NCLEX item type: multiple choice
Cognitive skill: compare
28. A patient asks the nurse how much exercise is considered enough for the control of blood pressure. The nurse knows that a range of 4–9 mm Hg of approximate systolic pressure reduction can occur with engaging in regular physical activity how often? *(356)*
    1. For as little as 30 minutes a week
    2. For at least 40 minutes 3–4 days a week
    3. For 15–20 minutes a week at the most
    4. For as little as 90 minutes a week
NCLEX item type: multiple choice
Cognitive skill: interpret
29. The nurse was instructing the patient in the scenario regarding lifestyle modification and recognized that further education was needed after the patient made which statement? *(355-356)*
    1. "So my plan is to start losing weight gradually so I can keep it off."
    2. "I know that I will have to stop eating tortilla chips since they have a lot of salt."
    3. "I understand that I need to walk more than just twice a week, so I think I will walk four times a week."
    4. "Since I will be started on drug therapy for my high blood pressure, I do not need to change my habits."
NCLEX item type: multiple choice
Cognitive skill: knowledge
30. While discussing the best way to change diet habits with a patient who has hypertension, the nurse asks the patient which appropriate question? *(360)*
    1. "Have you ever tried to adjust your portion size and number of servings from refined carbohydrates and sodium?"
    2. "Do you understand what is meant by restricting the amount of dairy products in your diet?"
    3. "Do you know how to estimate the percentage of total daily calories from fats?"
    4. "How is food prepared in the home? Do you prefer fried or baked foods?"
NCLEX item type: multiple choice
Cognitive skill: explain
31. A patient in scenario #1 was discussing how to manage his blood pressure with the nurse and mentioned that he likes to smoke an occasional cigar. What is the best response from the nurse? *(361)*
    1. "How often would you say is 'occasional'?"
    2. "That should be okay; smoking does not affect your blood pressure."
    3. "You will need to stop smoking altogether, since that is very bad for you."
    4. "Did you know that smoking will cause the diuretic you are on to be ineffective?"

Copyright © 2023 by Elsevier, Inc. All rights reserved.

Objective: Identify initial options and progression of medicines used to treat hypertension.
NCLEX item type: multiple response
Cognitive skill: classify
32. The nurse expects that the patient in scenario #1 may be started on which drug class? *(Select all that apply.)* **(356)**
    1. Thiazide diuretics
    2. Beta-adrenergic blockers
    3. Calcium channel blockers
    4. Aldosterone receptor antagonists
    5. Angiotensin-converting enzyme inhibitors
NCLEX item type: multiple choice
Cognitive skill: compare
33. After being on a thiazide for several months, the patient in scenario #2 being treated for stage 1 hypertension will most likely have which medication added because the target blood pressure was not attained? **(356)**
    1. aliskiren (Tekturna)
    2. eplerenone (Inspra)
    3. nifedipine (Procardia)
    4. spironolactone (Aldactone)
NCLEX item type: cloze
Cognitive skill: recognize cues
34. **Choose the most likely options for the information missing from the statements below by selecting from the list of options provided.**
    The nurse recognizes that for patients who have stage 2 hypertension there may be a progression of blood pressure control and a need to be started on two-drug combinations for blood pressure control, the two first line agents could be _____1_____./_____2_____ and _____1_____/_____2_____.**(356)**

Option 1	Option 2
Thiazide diuretics	Angiotensin II receptor blockers
Angiotensin-converting enzyme inhibitors	Calcium channel blockers
Angiotensin II receptor blockers	Thiazide diuretics
Calcium channel blockers	Angiotensin-converting enzyme inhibitors

Objective: Identify and summarize the action of five drug classes used to treat hypertension.
NCLEX item type: multiple choice
Cognitive skill: knowledge
35. The nurse recognizes the class of antihypertensive agents that lower blood pressure by blocking a very potent vasoconstrictor from binding to the receptor sites in vascular smooth muscle, brain, heart, kidneys, and adrenal glands as which class? **(367)**
    1. Beta blockers
    2. Angiotensin II receptor blockers

3. Calcium channel blockers
4. Aldosterone receptor antagonists
NCLEX item type: multiple choice
Cognitive skill: compare
36. The nurse needs to teach patients who develop a chronic, dry, nonproductive cough and are taking an antihypertensive agent, that they will need to contact their healthcare provider to get a different agent. Which medication would be likely to cause this adverse effect? **(365-366)**
    1. metoprolol
    2. hydralazine
    3. captopril
    4. amlodipine
NCLEX item type: multiple response
Cognitive skill: analyze
37. The nurse knows that calcium channel blockers are used for the reduction of blood pressure and have what other effect? *(Select all that apply.)* **(372-373)**
    1. Reduce the afterload of the heart
    2. Peripheral vasodilating effects
    3. Increase the sodium excretion in the kidneys
    4. Increase the preload of the heart
    5. Peripheral vasoconstricting effects
NCLEX item type: multiple response
Cognitive skill: application
38. The nurse discusses with a patient starting on the drug prazosin, an alpha-1 adrenergic blocking agent, and explains that the drug has which therapeutic effects? *(Select all that apply.)* **(375)**
    1. Improving memory
    2. Reducing blood lipids
    3. Improving urine flow
    4. Reducing blood pressure
    5. Reducing gastric acid production
NCLEX item type: multiple choice
Cognitive skill: explain
39. The nurse explains to the patient receiving hydralazine the effect the drug will have. Which statement by the nurse needs to be revised? **(378-379)**
    1. "Hydralazine is a direct vasodilator that results in a reduced peripheral vascular resistance."
    2. "This drug needs to be given with a beta blocker to prevent the reflex tachycardia that occurs."
    3. "Hydralazine is considered a first-line antihypertensive agents."
    4. "When you are on this drug you need to be aware that it may cause orthostatic hypotension."

Copyright © 2023 by Elsevier, Inc. All rights reserved.

Drugs Used to Treat Dysrhythmias

Answer Key: Textbook page references are provided as a guide for answering these questions. A complete answer key is provided to your instructor.

MATCHING

Match the term on the right with the definition on the left.

Definition

1. _____ an obstruction of conduction pathways, resulting in delayed conduction

2. _____ a disturbance in the normal electrical conduction of the heart, resulting in abnormal heart muscle contraction

3. _____ ringing in the ears

4. _____ digoxin

5. _____ a type of supraventricular dysrhythmia

6. _____ the electrical system of the heart

7. _____ the pacemaker cells in the conduction system

8. _____ dyspnea, chest pain, fatigue, edema, syncope, and palpitations

Term

a. conduction system
b. this antidysrhythmic agent works by slowing the conduction through the AV node
c. dysrhythmia
d. atrioventricular blocks
e. SA node
f. six cardinal signs of cardiovascular disease
g. paroxysmal supraventricular tachycardia (PSVT)
h. tinnitus

REVIEW QUESTIONS

Scenario: An 89-year-old patient was admitted to the hospital after falling and fracturing their arm. The patient has a history of atrial fibrillation and had a permanent pacemaker implanted several years ago.

Objective: Identify the classification of drugs used to treat dysrhythmias.

NCLEX item type: multiple response
Cognitive skill: explain

9. The nurse reviews with the patient in scenario #1 what the goals are for the treatment of dysrhythmias. Which statements by the nurse explain the goals? (*Select all that apply*.) *(383)*
   1. "An important goal for treating dysrhythmias is to speed up the heart rate."
   2. "An important goal for treating dysrhythmias is to restore normal sinus rhythm."
   3. "An important goal for treating dysrhythmias is to increase the contractility of the heart muscle."
   4. "An important goal for treating dysrhythmias is to prevent recurrence of life-threatening dysrhythmias."
   5. "An important goal for treating dysrhythmias is to improve the output from the atrial muscle."

NCLEX item type: multiple choice
Cognitive skill: classify

10. Of the medications that the patient in scenario #1 is taking, the nurse recognizes which medication for the treatment of atrial fibrillation? *(395)*
    1. irbasartan (Avapro)
    2. tramadol (Ultram)
    3. omeprazole (Prilosec)
    4. digoxin (Lanoxin)

Copyright © 2023 by Elsevier, Inc. All rights reserved.

NCLEX item type: drag and drop
Cognitive skill: evaluate cues
11. The nurse reviews the mechanism of action for the various classes of dysrhythmics.
    Indicate with an arrow which class corresponds with which mechanism of action. *(383-384)*

Classification of dysrhythmics	Mechanism of action
Class Ia agents	Prolongs the action potential of atrial and ventricular tissue and increased the refractory period
Class Ib agents	Inhibit cardiac response by blocking the L-type calcium channels in the SA and AV nodes
Class Ic agents	Potent myocardial depressants that slow the conduction rate through the atria and ventricles
Class II agents	Inhibit sodium ion movement in the myocardium
Class III agents	Inhibit cardiac response to sympathetic nerve stimulation by blocking the beta receptors
Class IV agents	Shorten the duration of the electrical stimulation and the time between electrical impulses

NCLEX item type: multiple choice
Cognitive skill: comprehension
12. The nurse knows that the class of antidysrhythmic drugs that is effective in inhibiting cardiac response to sympathetic nerve stimulation, and as a result, reduces heart rate, blood pressure, and cardiac output, is which type of agent? *(389)*
    1. Calcium channel blockers
    2. Beta-adrenergic blockers
    3. Potassium channel blockers
    4. Sodium channel blockers

Objective: Identify baseline nursing assessments that should be implemented during the treatment of dysrhythmias.
NCLEX item type: multiple response
Cognitive skill: application
13. Which methods does the nurse use to assess dysrhythmias that patients develop? *(Select all that apply.)* *(384)*
    1. Checking laboratory values
    2. Administering electric shock therapy
    3. Monitoring exercise treadmill results
    4. Interpreting electrocardiogram (ECG) readings
    5. Reviewing electrophysiologic studies (EPS)
NCLEX item type: multiple choice
Cognitive skill: analyze
14. The nurse recognizes that it is important to monitor the hourly urine output in a patient with dysrhythmias because this may indicate what? *(386)*
    1. The function of the atrial muscle
    2. The patient's degree of exercise tolerance
    3. Whether the kidneys are being adequately perfused
    4. Whether the peripheral tissues are being adequately perfused

NCLEX item type: multiple choice
Cognitive skill: interpret
15. Assessing a cardiac patient for level of consciousness is one of the important baseline assessments that the nurse will perform to determine if there is adequate what? *(385)*
    1. Peripheral perfusion
    2. Cerebral perfusion
    3. Renal perfusion
    4. Lung perfusion
Scenario #2: After suffering an out of hospital cardiac arrest the patient was diagnosed with ventricular tachycardia and started on an antiarrhythmic. The patient has a history of atrial flutter and currently takes aspirin and digoxin.

Objective: Discuss common adverse effects that may be observed with the administration of antidysrhythmic drugs.
NCLEX item type: multiple choice
Cognitive skill: comprehension
16. The patient in scenario #2 was given intravenously amiodarone to control the arrhythmia. The nurse will need to administer amiodarone by which method? *(390)*
    1. Infuse slowly over an hour, and flushed immediately
    2. Infuse slowly over an hour, then followed with a continuous drip
    3. Infuse quickly over 10 minutes, then flushed immediately
    4. Infuse quickly over 10 minutes, then followed with a continuous drip

Copyright © 2023 by Elsevier, Inc. All rights reserved.

NCLEX item type: multiple response
Cognitive skill: compare

17. The nurse needs to monitor which vital signs of patients who are taking antidysrhythmic drugs? (*Select all that apply.*) **(385)**
    1. Respirations
    2. Pulse quality
    3. Oxygen saturation
    4. Adequate intake
    5. Blood pressure in both arms

NCLEX item type: multiple response
Cognitive skill: interpret

18. The laboratory tests that the nurse should be monitored for the patient in scenario #1 taking an antidysrhythmic drug for atrial fibrillation include which values? (*Select all that apply.*) **(386)**
    1. Gastric pH
    2. Electrolytes
    3. Thyroid levels
    4. Arterial blood gases
    5. Creatine kinase (CK-MB)

NCLEX item type: multiple response
Cognitive skill: application

19. The nurse caring for a patient taking amiodarone knows that it may cause serious adverse effects, and the patient will need periodic tests to determine any effect on which bodily functions? (*Select all that apply.*) **(391)**
    1. Hearing loss
    2. Thyroid function
    3. Liver function
    4. Visual disturbance
    5. Pulmonary function

NCLEX item type: multiple response
Cognitive skill: explain

20. The nurse is teaching the patient in scenario #1 starting on propafenone (Rythmol SR) for further control of atrial fibrillation. The nurse teaches the patient to be alert for which common adverse effects of the drug? (*Select all that apply.*) **(389)**
    1. Tremors
    2. Dizziness
    3. Constipation
    4. Nausea and vomiting
    5. Sleep disturbances

NCLEX item type: extended multiple response
Cognitive skill: take action

21. When assessing the patient in scenario #2 who is taking flecainide, and currently stabilized on a dose of digoxin, the nurse observes for which signs and reports to the healthcare provider? (*Select all that apply.*) **(388)**
    1. Fatigue
    2. Respiratory depression
    3. Blurred or colored vision
    4. Bleeding gums and bruises
    5. Bradycardia
    6. Anorexia and nausea
    7. Tinnitus

Objective: Summarize the six cardinal signs of cardiovascular disease.

NCLEX item type: multiple choice
Cognitive skill: knowledge

22. The nurse assesses the patient in scenario #2 for which cardinal sign of cardiovascular disease that involves the respiratory system? **(384-385)**
    1. Dyspnea
    2. Palpitations
    3. Edema
    4. Syncope

NCLEX item type: multiple choice
Cognitive skill: illustrate

23. The patient in scenario #2 began complaining of feeling tired easily and starting to take naps in the afternoon. Which statement by the nurse is the most appropriate response? **(384-385)**
    1. "Your fatigue is just a matter of being in the hospital and not being as active as you are used to."
    2. "With your known cardiac history this fatigue is one of the signs of cardiovascular disease that we watch for to teach you what to expect."
    3. "You have a cardiac condition that caused an irregular heartbeat so your body is telling you to rest."
    4. "You will soon snap out of this feeling of fatigue in a few more days."

NCLEX item type: multiple response
Cognitive skill: compare

24. When monitoring patients for signs of cardiovascular disease, the nurse will observe for peripheral edema. Where are the specific areas of the body most likely to show signs of edema? (*Select all that apply.*) **(385)**
    1. Arms
    2. Mid-calf
    3. Ankles
    4. Thigh
    5. Hands

NCLEX item type: multiple choice
Cognitive skill: knowledge

25. The patient in the scenario told the nurse that he felt as though his heart was skipping some beats. The nurse recognized this symptom as which one of the six cardinal signs of cardiovascular disease? **(385)**
    1. Dyspnea
    2. Syncope
    3. Fatigue
    4. Palpitations

Copyright © 2023 by Elsevier, Inc. All rights reserved.

Drugs Used to Treat Angina Pectoris

Answer Key: Textbook page references are provided as a guide for answering these questions. A complete answer key is provided to your instructor.

MATCHING

Match the term on the right with the definition on the left.

Definition

1. _____   occurs while the patient is at rest, caused by vasospasms of the coronary artery, diagnosed by combination of history and exercise testing

2. _____   precipitated by physical exertion or stress, lasts only a few minutes, relieved by nitroglycerin

3. _____   unpredictable chest pain; changes in onset, frequency, duration, and intensity

4. _____   supply of oxygen needed by the heart cells is inadequate

5. _____   feeling of chest discomfort arising from the heart

Term

a.   unstable angina
b.   ischemia
c.   chronic stable angina
d.   angina pectoris
e.   variant angina

REVIEW QUESTIONS

Scenario: A 52-year-old male patient was admitted through the emergency department to a telemetry unit after experiencing sudden substernal chest pain radiating down his left arm. He complains of indigestion and indicates feeling faint. He was a history of urinary retention, palpitations, insomnia, and depression.

Objective: Discuss angina pectoris and identify assessment data needed to evaluate an anginal attack.

NCLEX item type: multiple choice
Cognitive skill: explain

6. The nurse educates the patient in scenario #1 on the underlying cause of anginal pain, which is a result of what? **(397)**
   1. A cardiac dysrhythmia
   2. A severe increase in blood pressure
   3. Decreased circulation to the chest muscles
   4. The lack of an adequate oxygen supply to the cells in the heart

NCLEX item type: multiple choice
Cognitive skill: application

7. The patient in scenario #1 has various presenting symptoms of angina, in addition to the substernal chest pain radiating down his left arm. Which symptoms will the nurse assess for that indicate ? *(Select all that apply.)* **(399)**
   1. Palpitations
   2. Depression
   3. Insomnia
   4. Feeling faint
   5. Urinary retention

NCLEX item type: multiple response
Cognitive skill: analyze

8. The nurse needs to gather which initial assessment data from the patient in scenario #1 who presents with angina? *(Select all that apply.)* **(389-399)**
   1. Any smoking history
   2. What medications are being taken
   3. Vital signs and pulse checks
   4. The onset, duration, and intensity of pain
   5. The degree of understanding regarding lifestyle modifications

Copyright © 2023 by Elsevier, Inc. All rights reserved.

Objective: Differentiate between *chronic stable angina* and *unstable angina*.
NCLEX item type: multiple choice
Cognitive skill: knowledge
9. The nurse recognized that the patient in scenario #1 is considered to have which type of angina? *(397)*
   1. Variant angina
   2. Unstable angina
   3. Chronic angina
   4. Stable angina
NCLEX item type: multiple choice
Cognitive skill: compare
10. The patient asks the nurse to explain the difference between unstable angina and chronic stable angina. Which statement by the nurse is accurate *(397)*
   1. "Chronic angina is relieved with rest and unstable angina is relieved with exercise."
   2. "Unstable angina is caused by vasospasm and chronic angina is caused by a fixed obstruction."
   3. "Chronic angina is unpredictable in nature and unstable angina occurs at regular intervals."
   4. "Unstable angina is relieved with nitroglycerin and chronic angina is relieved with statin drugs."
NCLEX item type: multiple response
Cognitive skill: relate
11. The nurse explaining to the patient in scenario #1 the treatment goals for angina will include which statements in the discussion? *(Select all that apply.)* *(397-398)*
   1. "The choices you have for treatment therapies are designed to prevent a heart attack."
   2. "Your healthcare team wants to improve quality of life by relieving your anginal pain."
   3. "You may have the choice of either angioplasty or bypass surgery depending on the results of further tests."
   4. "Depending on the results of your tests, you will be instructed to make changes in your lifestyle prior to starting on any drug therapy."
   5. "In the future, when you have anginal pain, you can take a Tylenol first before taking any nitroglycerin."

Scenario #2: A patient with a history of coronary artery disease who has chronic stable angina comes to the clinic for a routine physical checkup and after having an echocardiogram was started on an additional treatment to prevent ischemic attacks. The patient also has a history of diabetes, hypertension, dyslipidemia, and COPD.

Objective: Describe the actions and the adverse effects of the drug classifications used to treat angina.
NCLEX item type: multiple response
Cognitive skill: application
12. The nurse will perform which premedication assessments for the patient in scenario #1 prior to administering nitrates? *(Select all that apply.)* *(401)*
   1. Any history of gastritis
   2. The location, duration, and pattern of pain
   3. When the most recent nitrate was used
   4. Checking laboratory results of HDLs
   5. The ability to place the medication under the tongue correctly
NCLEX item type: multiple response
Cognitive skill: compare
13. The nurse expects the desired action of calcium channel blockers in the treatment of angina is to have what effect? *(Select all that apply.)* *(404)*
   1. Decrease myocardial oxygen demand
   2. Decrease resistance to blood flow
   3. Decrease the peripheral circulation
   4. Dilate the peripheral blood vessels
   5. Increase myocardial blood supply via coronary arteries
NCLEX item type: extended multiple response
Cognitive skill: recognize cues
14. The nurse expects that angiotensin-converting enzyme inhibitors used for the treatment of cardiovascular disease are used because they will have which actions? *(Select all that apply.)* *(405)*
   1. Promote vasodilation
   2. Induce tachypnea
   3. Minimize platelet aggregation
   4. Prevent hypotension
   5. Effect the walls of coronary arteries
   6. Inhibit urinary retention
   7. Reduce tinnitus
   8. Prevent thrombus formation

Copyright © 2023 by Elsevier, Inc. All rights reserved.

NCLEX item type: cloze
Cognitive skill: evaluate cues
Choose the most likely options for the information missing from the statements below by selecting from the list of options provided.

15. The nurse instructs the patient in scenario #2 regarding the medications from the drug class _____1_____ that needs to be observed closely in patients who have the diagnosis of_____2_____. *(404)*

Option 1	Option 2
ACE inhibitors	Anemia
Calcium channel blockers	COPD
Angiotensin receptor blockers	Hypertension
Beta-adrenergic blockers	Gastric ulcer

NCLEX item type: multiple response
Cognitive skill: application

16. The nurse administering nitrates to the patient in scenario #1 knows they are used for treatment of angina have they have which therapeutic outcomes? *Select all that apply. (401)*
    1. Cause the relief of anginal pain during an attack
    2. Prevent platelet aggregation
    3. Lower the amount of circulating LDLs
    4. Reduce the frequency and severity of anginal attacks
    5. Increased tolerance of activity

NCLEX item type: multiple choice
Cognitive skill: compare

17. The nurse reviews the mechanism of action for ACE inhibitors which are effective in relieving anginal attacks because they have which effect? *(405)*
    1. Prolong the QT interval
    2. Decrease serum creatinine
    3. Stabilize the sodium channels in myocardium
    4. Promote vasodilation and minimize platelet aggregation

NCLEX item type: multiple choice
Cognitive skill: explain

18. When educating the patient in scenario #2 regarding the calcium channel blocker diltiazem the nurse explains the actions of the drug. Which statement by the nurse is correct? *(404)*
    1. "The medication you are on, diltiazem will prevent platelet aggregation."
    2. " It is part of the properties of calcium channel blockers to lower the amount of circulating LDLs."
    3. "Calcium channel blockers such as diltiazem have the effect of increasing calcium levels in the blood."
    4. " An important effect that diltiazem does is dilate the peripheral vessels and inhibit smooth muscle contractions."

Objective: Discuss risk factor management and healthy lifestyle changes that are taught to prevent disease progression and myocardial infarction or death.
NCLEX item type: extended multiple response
Cognitive skill: evaluate cues

19. The nurse will teach the patient in scenario #2 lifestyle modifications that will include which recommendations? *Select all that apply. (400)*
    1. Report poor pain control to the healthcare provider
    2. Allow alcohol when taking nitrates
    3. Limit sexual activity and social interaction
    4. Dietary recommendations include a low sodium diet and to maintain ideal weight
    5. Participate in regular exercise is essential
    6. Manage stress with relaxation techniques or meditation
    7. Push to attain the degree of activity hoped for with drug therapy

NCLEX item type: multiple response
Cognitive skill: analyze

20. In addition to weight control and a structured exercise program, the nurse should also educate the patient in scenario #2 on other ways of improving cardiovascular health such as managing which conditions? *(Select all that apply.) (398)*
    1. Migraines
    2. Dyslipidemia
    3. Hypertension
    4. Hypothyroidism
    5. Diabetes mellitus

NCLEX item type: multiple response
Cognitive skill: application

21. The nurse was explaining to the patient in scenario #1 about the need to avoid activities that precipitate attacks of angina, which may include what examples? *(Select all that apply.) (397)*
    1. Watching TV
    2. Eating a light lunch
    3. Lifting heavy boxes
    4. Climbing a flight of stair
    5. Exposure to cold temperatures

Copyright © 2023 by Elsevier, Inc. All rights reserved.

Drugs Used to Treat Peripheral Vascular Disease

Answer Key: Textbook page references are provided as a guide for answering these questions. A complete answer key is provided to your instructor.

MATCHING
Match the term on the right with the definition on the left.

Definition

1. _____ a condition caused by vasospasms of the blood vessels triggered by unknown mechanisms

2. _____ numbness with a tingling sensation

3. _____ vasoconstriction of blood vessels

4. _____ pain secondary to lack of oxygen to the muscles during exercise

5. _____ obstructive arterial disease resulting from atherosclerotic plaque formation

Term

a. peripheral arterial disease
b. intermittent claudication
c. paresthesias
d. Raynaud disease
e. vasospasm

REVIEW QUESTIONS

Scenario #1: An 81-year-old male patient was admitted to the hospital with complaints of progressive pain in both legs with activity that no longer goes away when the activity is stopped.

Objective: Describe the baseline assessments needed to evaluate a patient with peripheral vascular disease.

NCLEX item type: multiple choice
Cognitive skill: comprehension

6. When caring for patients starting on vasodilating agents the nurse needs to assess for what adverse effect? *(410)*
   1. Paresthesias
   2. Pulsus paradoxus
   3. Orthostatic hypotension
   4. Thrombus formation

NCLEX item type: multiple choice
Cognitive skill: knowledge

7. The nurse explains to the patient in scenario #1 the most common form of peripheral vascular disease is knows as what? *(409)*
   1. Arteritis
   2. Obstructive arterial disease
   3. Raynaud's disease
   4. Coarctation of the aorta

NCLEX item type: multiple response
Cognitive skill: application

8. Baseline assessments the nurse will gather on the patient in scenario #1 regarding peripheral vascular disease include which factors? *(Select all that apply.)* *(411)*
   1. Limb pain
   2. Skin temperature
   3. Respiratory rate
   4. Peripheral pulses
   5. Presence of edema

NCLEX item type: multiple response
Cognitive skill: evaluate cues

9. The patient in scenario #1 has symptoms that may indicate intermittent claudication that is progressing. The nurse would expect which findings as further evidence of arteriosclerosis? *(Select all that apply.)* *(409)*
   1. Paresthesias
   2. Capillary refill of less than 3 seconds
   3. Poor pulses in the feet
   4. Waxy, pale, dry skin
   5. Cooler skin temperature of the legs

Copyright © 2023 by Elsevier, Inc. All rights reserved.

Objective: Identify specific measures that the patient can use to improve peripheral circulation and prevent the complications of peripheral vascular disease.

NCLEX item type: multiple choice
Cognitive skill: explain

10. Which statement by the nurse explains to patients with peripheral vascular disease why they should not elevate their extremities above the level of the heart? *(412)*
    1. "If you have your legs higher than your heart, the blood may tend to get too thin and cause problems."
    2. "It is important to not elevate your legs above the level of the heart since this will impair circulation."
    3. "Elevating your legs higher than your heart will cause vasospasms and aggravate the problem."
    4. "If your legs are above the level of your heart, it will make your heart work harder and you will get heart failure."

NCLEX item type: multiple response
Cognitive skill: application

11. The nurse explains to the patient in scenario #2 the most cost-effective and successful forms of treatment for peripheral vascular disease. Which examples does the nurse use to explain this? *(Select all that apply.)* *(410)*
    1. Exercise
    2. Medications
    3. Weight reduction
    4. Smoking cessation
    5. Dietary modification

NCLEX item type: grid/matrix
Cognitive skill: evaluate outcomes

12. The nurse educates the patient in scenario #2 on ways to improve peripheral circulation and prevent complications of peripheral vascular disease. *(412-413)*

Indicate with an 'X' in the correct column the recommendations for improving circulation and the ones used to prevent complications.

	Improves peripheral circulation	Prevent complications from peripheral vascular disease
Advise patient to avoid standing or sitting for prolonged periods		
Provide information about smoking cessation		
Advise patient not to cross knees or ankles		
Maintain adequate hydration		
Advise the patient to not elevate the extremities above the level of heart		
Instruct patient on medications used for vasodilation and inhibit platelet aggregation		
Monitor peripheral pulses; femoral, popliteal, and pedal		
Maintain meticulous foot and hand care		
Advise the patient not to go barefoot		
Avoid frostbite when exposed to cold temperatures		
Control obesity and blood lipid levels		

Scenario #2: 59-year-old patient came into the clinic complaining of pain in the legs during exercise, which has now caused some numbness. The healthcare provider has diagnoses the patient with intermittent claudication. The patient had a prescription written to help with the issue.

Copyright © 2023 by Elsevier, Inc. All rights reserved.

Objective: Identify treatment goals and what to expect when peripheral vasodilating agents are administered.

NCLEX item type: multiple choice
Cognitive skill: compare

13. Which agent that the patient in scenario #2 has been prescribed is approved by the FDA for treatment of intermittent claudication due to vasospasms? *(413)*
    1. Verapamil
    2. Clopidogrel
    3. Prazosin
    4. Cilostazol

NCLEX item type: multiple response
Cognitive skill: classify

14. The nurse researched the classes of drugs that are used for the treatment of intermittent claudication. Which ones does the nurse review? *(Select all that apply.) (410)*
    1. Direct vasodilators
    2. Calcium channel blockers
    3. Adrenergic antagonists
    4. Sodium channel blockers
    5. Angiotensin-converting enzyme inhibitors

NCLEX item type: cloze
Cognitive skill: recognizes cues

Choose the most likely options for the information missing from the statements below by selecting from the list of options provided.

15. The nurse expects that part of the treatment goals for the patient in scenario #2 would be ___1_____ and ___1___in addition, stressing to the patient that control of the diet, managing blood pressure, _2_____and __2_____will help met the goals. *(410)*

Option 1	Option 2
Increased mobility	Controlling diabetes
Improved blood flow	Reducing exposure to cold
Keeping feet warm	Continuing with current employment
Pain relief	Sleeping for 8 hours per night

NCLEX item type: multiple response
Cognitive skill: evaluate cues

16. A patient asks the nurse what can be done to decrease the occurrence and severity of vasospastic attacks of Raynaud disease. How does the nurse respond? *(Select all that apply.) (409-419)*
    1. "Most attacks of Raynaud disease can be stopped by avoiding hot temperatures."
    2. "Tobacco use is highly associated with vasospastic attacks of Raynaud disease."
    3. "It is not known what mechanisms trigger the vasospastic attacks seen with Raynaud disease."
    4. "The signs and symptoms associated with Raynaud disease are due to vasospasm of the arteries of the skin of the hands, fingers, and sometimes toes."
    5. "Most people have Raynaud disease for a few years and then it goes away."

Objective: Explain why hypotension and tachycardia occur frequently with the use of cilostazol.

NCLEX item type: multiple choice
Cognitive skill: illustrate

17. Because certain medications used for the treatment of peripheral vascular disease cause vasodilation, the nurse will need to instruct the patient to do what to prevent side effects? *(413)*
    1. Rise slowly
    2. Cross their legs when sitting
    3. Drink four glasses of water daily
    4. Encourage a diet high in salt intake

NCLEX item type: multiple response
Cognitive skill: generate solutions

18. The nurse will give instructions for an individual with peripheral vascular disease that includes which recommendations? *(Select all that apply.) (412)*
    1. Reduce or totally quit smoking
    2. Elevate the extremities above the heart
    3. Use self-care measures to promote peripheral circulation
    4. Avoid standing or sitting for prolonged periods of time
    5. Encourage patient to wear tight-fitting anklets or socks

NCLEX item type: multiple choice
Cognitive skill: interpret

19. The nurse was discussing with the patient some of the options that the healthcare provider and patient had reviewed earlier in the day. To clarify the patient's options, the nurse could make which therapeutic statement? *(413)*
    1. "The provider talked to you about surgical options when you feel the medications are no longer effective."
    2. "The surgical options are the way to go and get this problem taken care of, in my opinion."
    3. "The provider said to you that amputation of your leg is the next step, rather than angioplasty or bypass grafting."
    4. "There is nothing further we can do for you. You will just have to suffer because there are no more options available to you other than the medications."

Copyright © 2023 by Elsevier, Inc. All rights reserved.

Drugs Used to Treat Thromboembolic Disorders

Answer Key: Textbook page references are provided as a guide for answering these questions. A complete answer key is provided to your instructor.

MATCHING
Match the term on the right with the definition on the left.

Definition

1. _____ drug class that inhibits platelet aggregation

2. _____ drug class that is active against factor Xa and thrombin

3. _____ triggered by sources outside the blood vessels, such as tissue extract or thromboplastin

4. _____ drug class that inhibits thrombin, preventing the conversion of fibrinogen to fibrin

5. _____ drug class that acts by blocking receptors on platelets, preventing clot formation

6. _____ a small fragment of a thrombus that breaks off

7. _____ drug class that causes the dissolution of fibrin clots

8. _____ a fibrin blood clot

9. _____ activated when a blood vessel is injured and collagen in the vessel wall is exposed

Term

a. thrombus
b. embolus
c. intrinsic clotting pathway
d. extrinsic clotting pathway
e. fibrinolytic agents
f. platelet inhibitors
g. anticoagulants
h. thrombin inhibitors
i. glycoprotein IIb/IIIa inhibitors

REVIEW QUESTIONS

Scenario #1: An 82-year-old patient was admitted to the hospital with a stroke. The patient has a history of atrial fibrillation and noncompliance with medications.

Objective: Describe conditions that place an individual at risk for developing blood clots and nursing interventions used to prevent these conditions.

NCLEX item type: multiple response
Cognitive skill: application

10. The nurse recognizes that certain conditions put patients at risk for developing blood clots. Which patient conditions will the nurse recognize as potential risks? *(Select all that apply.)* **(417)**
   1. Pulmonary embolism
   2. Certain types of cancers
   3. Pregnancy and oral contraceptives
   4. Immobilization or trauma of the lower limbs
   5. Surgery and postoperative period

NCLEX item type: multiple response
Cognitive skill: interpret

11. The nurse recognizes that the patient in scenario #1 is at risk for developing a clot that breaks off and creates a pulmonary embolism because of what factors? *(Select all that apply.)* **(419)**
   1. The patient is noncompliant with medications.
   2. The patient is taking medications on a regular basis.
   3. The patient has atrial fibrillation, which is known to cause blood clots.
   4. The patient walks slowly because of advanced age and it slows the blood flow.
   5. The healthcare provider had not prescribed the correct medications to prevent a blood clot.

Copyright © 2023 by Elsevier, Inc. All rights reserved.

NCLEX item type: multiple response
Cognitive skill: application
12. The nurse will perform which nursing actions to help prevent the formation of a clot in those patients who are at risk for developing blood clots? *(Select all that apply.)* **(418)**
    1. Restrict fluid intake to 1 liter/day.
    2. Assess perfusion of extremities.
    3. Flex the patient's knees when on bedrest.
    4. Administering anticoagulants as ordered
    5. Apply sequential compression devices as prescribed by the healthcare provider.

NCLEX item type: multiple response
Cognitive skill: analyze
13. The nurse knows which types of patients are at risk for developing clots? *(Select all that apply.)* **(419)**
    1. Patients who are on prolonged bedrest
    2. Patients who have had a history of blood clots
    3. Patients who limit their intake of green leafy vegetables
    4. Patients who have recently had orthopedic or thoracic surgery
    5. Patient who are adequately controlled on anticoagulation therapy

Objective: Identify the actions of platelet inhibitors, anticoagulants, thrombin inhibitors, and fibrinolytic agents.

NCLEX item type: cloze
Cognitive skill: recognize cues
Choose the most likely options for the information missing from the statements below by selecting from the list of options provided.
14. The nurse knows the primary purpose of anticoagulants such as __1__ administered after a blood clot is discovered is to __2__. **(418)**

Option 1	Option 2
aspirin	prevent the clot from forming
clopidogrel	decrease the size of the clot
warfarin	dissolve the existing clot
dabigatran	prevent the extension of the existing clot

NCLEX item type: multiple choice
Cognitive skill: knowledge
15. The nurse knows that when a small fragment of a thrombus breaks off and circulates until it becomes trapped causing a cerebral embolism, the treatment of choice would be to use what class of drug? **(424)**
    1. Anticoagulant
    2. Thrombin inhibitor
    3. Platelet inhibitor
    4. Fibrinolytic agent

NCLEX item type: extended multiple response
Cognitive skill: recognize cues
16. The nurse explains to the patient in scenario #1 that there are medications used to prevent clot formation for patients with atrial fibrillation. Which drugs would the nurse expect the patient to be prescribed? **(424,432)**
    1. aspirin
    2. clopidogrel
    3. prasugrel
    4. apixaban
    5. dalteparin
    6. warfarin

NCLEX item type: multiple response
Cognitive skill: generate solutions
17. When patients are receiving anticoagulant therapy, the nurse should instruct them on which measures to prevent clot formation? *(Select all that apply.)* **(420)**
    1. Regular ambulation
    2. Not to flex the knees
    3. Active or passive leg exercises
    4. Placing pressure against the popliteal space behind the knees
    5. Standing or sitting motionless for prolonged periods of time

NCLEX item type: multiple choice
Cognitive skill: compare
18. The nurse recognizes that the thrombin inhibitor dabigatran (Pradaxa) has which major advantage over anticoagulants used for reducing the risk of stroke or systemic embolism? **(434)**
    1. When metabolized, it takes the form of four active metabolites
    2. The capsules are taken two times daily with or without food
    3. The drug does not require monitoring of blood tests to adjust the dosage
    4. Baseline blood pressure readings need to be obtained supine and standing

Scenario # 2: A patient on the surgical floor recovering from orthopedic surgery was prescribed bedrest for two days. The nurse caring for the patient implemented nursing cares to prevent post-operative complications.

Objective: Describe specific monitoring procedures and laboratory data used to detect hemorrhage in the patient taking anticoagulants.

NCLEX item type: multiple response
Cognitive skill: take action
19. Which premedication assessments should be performed by the nurse before administering aspirin as a platelet inhibitor? *(Select all that apply.)* **(421)**
    1. Monitor serum potassium levels
    2. Perform a neurologic assessment
    3. Observe for any gastrointestinal symptoms
    4. Determine any concurrent use of antihypertensives
    5. Get a baseline serum glucose if on oral hypoglycemic

Copyright © 2023 by Elsevier, Inc. All rights reserved.

NCLEX item type: multiple choice
Cognitive skill: interpret

20. What therapeutic response does the nurse need to monitor when patients are on warfarin (Jantoven)? *(432)*
    1. Occult blood will be evident in stools.
    2. Urine may appear red, smoke-colored, or brownish.
    3. The prothrombin time (PT) or INR results will be within the recommended range.
    4. The skin and mucous membranes will have petechiae, ecchymosis, or hematomas.

NCLEX item type: multiple choice
Cognitive skill: illustrate

21. Which adverse effect from warfarin (Jantoven) does the nurse monitor for that indicates the patient is bleeding under the skin? *(433)*
    1. Anemia
    2. Petechiae
    3. Hematuria
    4. Thrombocytopenia

NCLEX item type: multiple response
Cognitive skill: application

22. A prescription for subcutaneous heparin for the patient in scenario #2 was received by the nurse, who will prepare and administer the drug after reviewing which precautions? *(Select all that apply.)* *(428)*
    1. Plan to use the abdominal area.
    2. Avoid rotating sites of injection.
    3. Obtain the correct needle length—usually 1/2 inch.
    4. Avoid an area of 2 inches around the umbilicus.
    5. After injecting the drug, massage the area for 10 seconds.

NCLEX item type: multiple response
Cognitive skill: evaluate outcomes

23. The nurse will observe for which specific events to detect for internal bleeding in patients on IV heparin? *(Select all that apply.)* *(429)*
    1. Paresthesias
    2. Increasing pulse
    3. Cold, clammy skin
    4. Decreasing blood pressure
    5. Disoriented sensorium

NCLEX item type: multiple choice
Cognitive skill: knowledge

24. When administering heparin, the nurse knows that this drug can be administered by which routes? *(428)*
    1. Orally, IM, IV
    2. Subcutaneously, IV
    3. IM, subcutaneously, IV
    4. Orally, subcutaneously, IV

Objective: Describe the nursing assessments needed to monitor therapeutic response and adverse effects from anticoagulant therapy.

NCLEX item type: multiple response
Cognitive skill: application

25. The therapeutic effect of heparin is monitored by the nurse with which laboratory tests? *(Select all that apply.)* *(428)*
    1. Protime
    2. Platelets
    3. aPTT
    4. Anti-factor Xa
    5. Hematocrit

NCLEX item type: multiple response
Cognitive skill: take action

26. Nurses will educate the patient in scenario #1 on what to report when on Jantoven therapy and include which symptoms, which may indicate a need to check the INR? *(Select all that apply.)* *(433)*
    1. Black tarry stools
    2. Nosebleeds
    3. Claudication
    4. Petechiae
    5. Coffee-ground or blood-tinged vomitus

NCLEX item type: multiple response
Cognitive skill: application

27. The nurse educates the patient taking apixaban (Eliquis) on which adverse effects that need to be reported? *(Select all that apply.)* *(426)*
    1. Ataxia
    2. Nystagmus
    3. Hematuria
    4. Easy bruising
    5. Black tarry stools

NCLEX item type: multiple choice
Cognitive skill: knowledge

28. What is the normal therapeutic range of INR that the nurse will monitor for warfarin (Jantoven) therapy on a patient with a mechanical prosthetic heart valve? *(432)*
    1. 1.5–2.0
    2. 2.0–3.0
    3. 2.5–3.5
    4. 3.0–3.5

Copyright © 2023 by Elsevier, Inc. All rights reserved.

Student Name_____ Date_____

Drugs Used to Treat Heart Failure

Answer Key: Textbook page references are provided as a guide for answering these questions. A complete answer key is provided to your instructor.

MATCHING
Match the definition on the right with the key term on the left.

Term

1. _____ heart failure with reduced ejection fractions

2. _____ positive inotropy

3. _____ inotropic agents

4. _____ digitalis toxicity

5. _____ negative chronotropy

6. _____ heart failure with preserved ejection fraction

Definition

a. having the ability to slow the heart rate

b. when the heart lacks sufficient force to pump all the blood

c. having the ability to stimulate the heart to increase the force of contractions

d. signs and symptoms include anorexia, nausea, and bradycardia

e. when the heart fails to relax enough between contractions to allow adequate filling

f. drugs that stimulate the heart to increase the force of contractions

REVIEW QUESTIONS
Scenario #1: An 88-year-old patient was admitted to the hospital with the diagnosis of exacerbation of heart failure. The patient has a history of coronary artery disease (CAD) with a stent placed in the past, hypertension, hyperlipidemia, diabetes, and asthma.

Objective: Explain heart failure in terms of the body's compensatory mechanisms.
NCLEX item type: multiple response
Cognitive skill: application
7. The patient in scenario #1 has symptoms of heart failure with reduced ejection fraction causing decreased cardiac output and decreased tissue perfusion. What can the nurse expect to find upon assessment? *(Select all that apply.)* *(438)*
   1. Poor peripheral perfusion
   2. Insomnia
   3. Bradypnea
   4. Tinnitus
   5. Exercise intolerance

NCLEX item type: multiple choice
Cognitive skill: knowledge
8. The nurse remembers that heart failure with preserved ejection fraction occurs because of what? *(438)*
   1. The peripheral vasculature develops stiffness.
   2. The symptoms of pulmonary embolism develop.
   3. The left ventricle becomes soft and boggy from being distended.
   4. The left ventricle becomes stiff and fails to relax, thus it does not fill adequately prior to the next contraction.

NCLEX item type: multiple choice
Cognitive skill: explain
9. The nurse understands that when patients are in heart failure, the kidneys respond to the decreased perfusion via the renin-angiotensin-aldosterone system, which stimulates the renal distal tubules to increase blood volume by what mechanism? *(439)*
   1. Excreting excess fluid
   2. Retaining sodium and water
   3. Increasing renin production
   4. Releasing epinephrine and norepinephrine

Objective: Identify the goals of treatment of heart failure.

NCLEX item type: multiple choice
Cognitive skill: knowledge

10. The nurse educates the patient in scenario #1 on their underlying diseases that are treated to correct the heart failure. Which patient conditions will be discussed by the nurse? *(Select all that apply.)* **(440)**
    1. Asthma
    2. Hyperlipidemia
    3. Hypertension
    4. Diabetes
    5. CAD

NCLEX item type: extended multiple response
Cognitive skill: recognize cues

11. The nurse discusses the goals of treatment for heart failure with the patient in scenario #1 and includes what outcomes in the discussion? *(Select all that apply.)* **(439)**
    1. Prolonging life
    2. Increasing intravascular volume
    3. Increasing exercise tolerance
    4. Reversing the ventricular damage
    5. Improving kidney function
    6. Improving quality of life
    7. Reducing signs and symptoms of fluid overload
    8. Being able to use only one drug to improve symptoms

NCLEX item type: multiple response
Cognitive skill: application

12. The patient in scenario #1 will be educated by the nurse on lifestyle changes that are aimed at improving heart failure. Which questions should the nurse ask of the patient to get them thinking about this? *(Select all that apply.)* **(445)**
    1. "What kinds of coping mechanisms do you use when you are stressed."
    2. "What do you do at home when you get short of breath? We need to discuss the proper way to position yourself during these times."
    3. "Are you currently keeping track of your blood pressure, pulse, and respirations at home?"
    4. "Do you space your activities of daily living in such a way that will conserve your energy and avoid fatigue."
    5. "Are you drinking plenty of water with your meals?"

Scenario #2: A 78 year-old patient who has been treated for many years for heart failure is now being started on digoxin. The patient also has a history of atrial fibrillation and hypothyroidism along with chronic kidney insufficiency.

Objective: Identify the primary actions on heart failure of digoxin, ACE inhibitors, ARBs, the combination of a neprilysin inhibitor with an ARB (Entresto), and beta blockers.

NCLEX item type: multiple response
Cognitive skill: application

13. The nurse explains to the patient in scenario #2 what the desired therapeutic outcomes of digoxin are for the treatment of heart failure. Which outcomes will the nurse mention in the discussion? *(Select all that apply.)* **(448-449)**
    1. Improvement of dyspnea
    2. Improved tolerance of activity
    3. Tolerating oxygen therapy during rest
    4. Maintaining a serum digoxin level of 2.0 ng/mL
    5. Improved cardiac output resulting in improved tissue perfusion

NCLEX item type: multiple choice
Cognitive skill: contrast

14. When angiotensin-converting enzyme (ACE) inhibitors are used primarily in heart failure the nurse understands they will have what effect? **(446)**
    1. They increase the secretion of aldosterone.
    2. They increase sodium excretion in the kidneys.
    3. They reduce afterload of the heart by blocking vasoconstriction.
    4. They stimulate the heart to increase the force of contractions.

NCLEX item type: multiple choice
Cognitive skill: compare

15. The nurse planning on administering a beta-adrenergic blocking agents for a heart failure patient understands that these drugs will have what effect? **(448)**
    1. They increase sodium excretion.
    2. They increase the secretion of aldosterone.
    3. They inhibit renin release to improve symptoms of heart failure.
    4. They stimulate the renin-angiotensin-aldosterone system.

Copyright © 2023 by Elsevier, Inc. All rights reserved.

NCLEX item type: multiple choice
Cognitive skill: illustrate
16. The patient in scenario #2 is starting on Entresto and asks the nurse what effect this will have on their heart failure. Which statement by the nurse is correct? *(446)*
    1. "The drug Entresto is a combination drug will increase vascular resistance to help with heart failure."
    2. "The combination drug Entresto is used in the treatment of heart failure and works to reduce preload and afterload."
    3. "The combination drug Entresto works by different mechanisms to slow the contractility of the heart."
    4. "The combination drug Entresto will reduce circulating blood volume by stimulating the secretion of aldosterone.

NCLEX item type: multiple choice
Cognitive skill: explain
17. The nurse read the chart from the patient in scenario #2 who had recently been in the ICU for short-term management of heart failure with a phosphodiesterase inhibitor milrinone given IV. The nurse remembered the actions of milrinone include what? *(Select all that apply.)* *(450)*
    1. Increases the force and velocity of myocardial contractions
    2. Inhibits cardiac response to nerve stimulation, reducing blood pressure
    3. Relaxes vascular smooth muscle which causes vasodilation
    4. Inhibits the cardiac pacemaker electrical current in the SA node, slowing heart rate
    5. Reduces preload and afterload of the heart

Objective: Describe digoxin toxicity and ways to prevent it.
NCLEX item type: multiple choice
Cognitive skill: interpret
18. When the patient in scenario #2 with heart failure on multiple medications starts to complain of loss of appetite with nausea as well as extreme fatigue, and nightmares, the nurse should consider that what may be happening? *(449)*
    1. The patient is having dysrhythmias.
    2. The patient is experiencing digoxin toxicity.
    3. The patient is noncompliant with medications.
    4. The patient is experiencing worsening of heart failure.

NCLEX item type: multiple response
Cognitive skill: taking action
19. The nurse knows that hypokalemia may induce digitalis toxicity. Monitoring the patient's potassium level is crucial to preventing digitalis toxicity as well as what other assessments or interventions will the nurse perform? *(Select all that apply.)* *(449-450)*
    1. Monitoring the digoxin level in the blood
    2. Monitoring the pulse oximeter level
    3. Knowing what the antidote is for digoxin toxicity
    4. Monitoring the heart rate for bradycardia
    5. Knowing what drugs may enhance the effect of digoxin

Objective: Identify essential assessment data and nursing interventions needed for a patient with heart failure.
NCLEX item type: multiple response
Cognitive skill: generate solutions
20. The nurse is teaching the patient in scenario #2 important health promotion measures and will emphasize which steps for the patient to take? *(Select all that apply.)* *(445)*
    1. Expect a short-term treatment
    2. Continue with a lifelong treatment
    3. Practice an exercise regimen
    4. Follow a diet low in sodium
    5. Manage your medications by understanding their purpose

NCLEX item type: multiple response
Cognitive skill: classify
21. The nurse reviewed the drug classes used to treat patients in Stage A heart failure. Which drug classes are included in the list for Stage A? *(Select all that apply.)* *(442)*
    1. Diuretics
    2. Statins
    3. Beta blockers
    4. ACE inhibitors
    5. Angiotensin II receptor blockers

Copyright © 2023 by Elsevier, Inc. All rights reserved.

NCLEX item type: grid/matrix
Cognitive skill: evaluate cues

22. The nurse reviewed the six cardinal signs of heart disease associated with inadequate tissue perfusion. *(442-444)* **Indicate with an 'X' the correct column the signs and symptoms are associated with. The symptoms are used only once.**

	Cardinal signs of heart disease	Common adverse cardiovascular effects from drugs	Cardiac dysrhythmias
Atrial fibrillation			
Palpitations			
Hyperkalemia			
Edema			
Syncope			
Chest pain			
Bradycardia			
Hypotension			
Dizziness			
Tachycardia			
Fatigue			
Dyspnea			

Copyright © 2023 by Elsevier, Inc. All rights reserved.

Drugs Used for Diuresis

Answer Key: Textbook page references are provided as a guide for answering these questions. A complete answer key is provided to your instructor.

MATCHING
Match the definition on the left with the key term on the right.

Definition

1. _____ a hormone that inhibits reabsorption of sodium in the distal tubule

2. _____ an excess of uric acid in the blood

3. _____ part of the kidney responsible for reabsorption of sodium and chloride

4. _____ dizziness, weakness, and faintness associated with a drop in blood pressure

5. _____ the part of the kidney tubule that forms a long loop in the medulla of the kidney

6. _____ a term used to describe excess fluid accumulation in the extracellular spaces

Term

a. edema
b. loop of Henle
c. aldosterone
d. hyperuricemia
e. tubule
f. orthostatic hypotension

REVIEW QUESTIONS

Scenario #1: A 74-year-old patient was admitted to the hospital with a recent urinary tract infection. It was subsequently found that the patient had hyponatremia, with an acute kidney injury and history of hypertension and heart failure. The patient was started on several medications to treat the underlying disorders and one of the drugs is a diuretic.

Objective: Identify the nursing assessments used to evaluate a patient's state of hydration and renal function.
NCLEX item type: multiple choice
Cognitive skill: knowledge

7. When assessing a patient who is overhydrated, which assessment finding does the nurse expect to see? *(456)*
   1. Poor skin turgor
   2. Deteriorating vital signs
   3. Deeply furrowed tongue
   4. Neck vein distention

NCLEX item type: multiple response
Cognitive skill: evaluate

8. What are the classic signs of dehydration that the nurse will assess for and report? *(Select all that apply.)* *(455)*
   1. Weak pedal pulses
   2. Soft or sunken eyeballs
   3. Delayed capillary filling
   4. Shrunken or deeply furrowed tongue

   5. Skin turgor elastic with rapid return to flat position

NCLEX item type: multiple response
Cognitive skill: interpret

9. The nurse knows that a patient who has received IV fluids in excess of fluids excreted is likely to develop which signs of overhydration? *(Select all that apply.)* *(456)*
   1. Peripheral edema around the ankles
   2. Presence of crackles in the lungs
   3. Sunken eyeballs
   4. Hypernatremia
   5. Mucous membranes that glisten

NCLEX item type: extended multiple response
Cognitive skill: recognize cues

10. When taking a history of a patient with fluid volume excess, the nurse should ask the patient questions relating to any history of heart disorders that contribute to fluid volume excess such as which conditions? *(Select all that apply.)* *(455)*
   1. Mitral stenosis
   2. Atrial fibrillation
   3. Supraventricular tachycardia
   4. Myocardial infarction
   5. Patent foramen ovale (PFO)
   6. Endocarditis
   7. Heart failure
   8. Aortic aneurysm

Copyright © 2023 by Elsevier, Inc. All rights reserved.

NCLEX item type: multiple response
Cognitive skill: application

11. The nurse should be aware of which types of susceptible people who are at risk for the development of electrolyte disturbances? *(Select all that apply.)* *(456)*
    1. Patients who are pregnant
    2. Patients with massive trauma
    3. Patients who are receiving steroid therapy
    4. Patients with a history of cardiac disease
    5. Patients with a history of hormonal disorders

NCLEX item type: multiple response
Cognitive skill: compare

12. The nurse needs to review laboratory studies for the patient in scenario #1 who had been prescribed diuretic therapy. Which laboratory values will the nurse monitor? *(Select all that apply.)* *(456)*
    1. BUN
    2. Sodium
    3. Potassium
    4. Creatinine
    5. Platelets

Scenario #2: A diabetic patient on an oral hypoglycemic agent comes into the hospital with heart failure for recent weight gain with +4 pitting edema. The patient was started on furosemide to diuresis excess fluid.

Objective: Describe the actions of diuretics and their effects on blood pressure and electrolytes.

NCLEX item type: multiple response
Cognitive skill: application

13. The nurse explains to the patient in scenario #1 what the therapeutic outcome is expected when patients are on diuretic therapy. Which statement by the nurse is incorrect? *(Select all that apply.)* *(454)*
    1. "Diuretic therapy will reduced the edema you have in your legs."
    2. "One of the results we are looking for with diuretic therapy is a decreased blood pressure."
    3. "When we give patients diuretics we expect that is will be only for a limited time."
    4. "Diuretic therapy is used to improve the symptoms of excess fluid volume, by allowing the kidneys to remove extra water from the body."
    5. "The therapeutic outcome from diuretics is a decreased excretory load on the kidneys."

NCLEX item type: multiple choice
Cognitive skill: evaluate

14. The patient in scenario #1 is currently taking digoxin (Lanoxin), aminoglycosides, nonsteroidal anti-inflammatory drugs (NSAIDs), and corticosteroids for multiple medical problems. Which principle does the nurse consider in monitoring this patient when bumetanide has now been prescribed? *(459-460)*
    1. The amount of digoxin will need to be increased.
    2. The potential for ototoxicity from the aminoglycosides is increased.
    3. The dose of bumetanide will need to be decreased when also taking NSAIDs.
    4. The use of corticosteroids and bumetanide may cause hyperkalemia.

NCLEX item type: multiple response
Cognitive skill: analyze

15. The patient in scenario #2 is being treated with metformin (Glucophage), warfarin (Jantoven), and digitalis. The patient has a new prescription for bumetanide (Bumex). What adverse effects does the nurse watch for? *(Select all that apply.)* *(459-460)*
    1. Edema
    2. Dry mouth
    3. Fluid overload
    4. Orthostatic hypotension
    5. Electrolyte imbalance

NCLEX item type: multiple response
Cognitive skill: application

16. The nurse administering thiazides to patients will monitor which electrolyte? *(Select all that apply.)* *(462)*
    1. Chloride (Cl−)
    2. Potassium (K+)
    3. Sodium (Na+)
    4. Magnesium (Mg+)
    5. Phosphorus (PO^{3-})
    6. Calcium (Ca+)

NCLEX item type: multiple choice
Cognitive skill: comprehension

17. The nurse knows that when thiazide diuretics such as chlorothiazide (Diuril) are administered, the drug is acting primarily on what part of the kidney? *(461)*
    1. The ascending limb of the loop of Henle
    2. The descending limb of the loop of Henle
    3. The distal tubules of the kidneys
    4. Enzymes in the kidneys that promote excretion of sodium and water

NCLEX item type: multiple choice
Cognitive skill: relate

18. When the nurse administers carbonic anhydrase inhibitors the drug can be used as a mild diuretic, and also as an effective agent for which condition? *(458)*
    1. Glaucoma
    2. Hypothyroidism
    3. Gouty arthritis
    4. Peripheral neuropathy

NCLEX item type: multiple response
Cognitive skill: application

19. The nurse recognizes potent diuretics that act primarily by inhibiting sodium and chloride reabsorption from the ascending limb of the loop of Henle in the kidneys include which drugs? *(Select all that apply.)* *(458)*
    1. bumetanide
    2. metolazone
    3. furosemide
    4. torsemide
    5. acetazolamide

Copyright © 2023 by Elsevier, Inc. All rights reserved.

Objective: Explain the rationale for administering diuretics cautiously to older adults and individuals with impaired renal function, cirrhosis of the liver, or diabetes mellitus.

NCLEX item type: multiple response
Cognitive skill: analyze

20. The patient in scenario #2 has the diagnosis of diabetes, and will most likely have to be supplemented with what? *(Select all that apply.)* *(459)*
    1. Potassium
    2. Oxygen
    3. Magnesium
    4. Extra oral hypoglycemic agents
    5. IV fluids

NCLEX item type: cloze
Cognitive skill: recognize cues

Choose the most likely options for the information missing from the statements below by selecting from the list of options provided.

21. The nurse knows that ethacrynic acid (Edecrin) is used to treat edema from _____1_____ and _____1_____. The patients taking Edecrin are at risk for developing _____2_____, _____2_____ and _____2_____with impaired renal function. *(460)*

Option 1	Option 2
Hyperglycemia	Mental confusion
Heart failure	Dizziness
Hyperuricemia	Diarrhea
Cirrhosis of the liver	Tinnitus
Hypersensitivity	Deafness

NCLEX item type: multiple response
Cognitive skill: interpret

22. The nurse discusses with the patient in scenario #1 the reasons for the medication furosemide (Lasix). Which statements by the nurse need to be corrected? *(Select all that apply.)* *(458)*
    1. "Lasix is the drug we give patients who have hypotension."
    2. "We are using the Lasix to treat your urinary tract infection."
    3. "This drug will induce hypernatremia to treat your hyponatremia."
    4. "The Lasix will help you get rid of excess fluid that your heart failure is causing."
    5. "Your hypertension and heart failure can be improved with the use of Lasix."

NCLEX item type: multiple response
Cognitive skill: application

23. The nurse explains to the patient who is on hydrochlorothiazide that it is used as a diuretic to reduce edema and improve symptoms associated with which conditions? *(Select all that apply.)* *(461)*
    1. Renal disease
    2. Hyperglycemia
    3. Heart failure
    4. Hepatic disease
    5. Premenstrual syndrome

NCLEX item type: multiple choice
Cognitive skill:

24. The nurse gives instructions to a patient who is on the potassium sparing diuretic spironolactone. Which statement by the nurse is incorrect? *(464)*
    1. "One of the adverse effects to watch for is headache, is one persists please report this to your healthcare provider."
    2. "This diuretic can be given with other diuretics to increase its effectiveness."
    3. "We will need to monitor your potassium while on this medication because it can cause hypokalemia."
    4. "If you take this medication with food or milk it should reduce any gastric irritation."

Objective: Identify the nursing assessments needed to monitor the therapeutic response or the development of common or serious adverse effects of diuretic therapy.

NCLEX item type: multiple response
Cognitive skill: application

25. When administering thiazide and loop diuretics to a diabetic patient, the nurse will need to monitor what lab results to prevent an adverse reaction? *(Select all that apply.)* *(462)*
    1. Sodium
    2. Potassium
    3. Blood sugar
    4. Hemoglobin
    5. Prothrombin time

NCLEX item type: multiple choice
Cognitive skill: knowledge

26. The nurse cautions the patients taking salt substitutes while on spironolactone (Aldactone), since the patient's laboratory results may indicate which electrolyte imbalance? *(463)*
    1. Hypokalemia
    2. Hyponatremia
    3. Hypercalcemia
    4. Hyperkalemia

Copyright © 2023 by Elsevier, Inc. All rights reserved.

NCLEX item type: multiple response
Cognitive skill: application

27. What premedication assessments should be performed by the nurse on patients prescribed triamterene (Dyrenium)? *(Select all that apply.)* **(465)**
    1. baseline weights
    2. blood pressure
    3. presence of edema
    4. electrolytes and renal labs
    5. need for hearing aids

NCLEX item type: grid/matrix
Cognitive skill: recognize cues

28. The nurse observes the patient for signs of adverse effects from diuretic therapy which include electrolyte imbalance. Indicate with an 'X' which symptom is from electrolyte imbalance and which is an adverse effect from diuretics. Each symptom is used only once. **(460)**

	Electrolyte imbalance symptoms	Adverse effects from diuretic therapy
Altered mental status		
Diarrhea		
Nocturia		
Nausea		
Muscle cramps		
Tremors		
Postural hypotension		

Copyright © 2023 by Elsevier, Inc. All rights reserved.

Drugs Used to Treat Upper Respiratory Disease

Answer Key: Textbook page references are provided as a guide for answering these questions. A complete answer key is provided to your instructor.

MATCHING

Match the definition on the left with the key term on the right.

Definition

1. _____ a rebound of nasal secretions caused from overuse of topical decongestants

2. _____ drugs of choice for relieving congestion associated with rhinitis caused by the common cold

3. _____ a compound derived from an amino acid stored in small granules in most body tissues

4. _____ an inflammation of the nasal mucosa

5. _____ an inflammation of the nasal mucosa as a result of an allergic reaction

6. _____ a runny nose from nasal and lacrimal secretions

7. _____ a drug class that works by competing with the allergy-liberated histamine for H_1 receptor sites

Key Term

a. histamine
b. allergic rhinitis
c. antihistamines
d. rhinorrhea
e. rhinitis medicamentosa
f. decongestants
g. rhinitis

REVIEW QUESTIONS

Scenario #1: A 48-year-old patient came into the clinic complaining of itchy, red eyes, and frequent sneezing with nasal congestion. The patient was diagnosed with allergic rhinitis.

Objective: Discuss the causes of allergic rhinitis and nasal congestion and rhinitis medicamentosa.

NCLEX item type: multiple response
Cognitive skill: analyze cues

8. The nurse explains to the patient in the scenario the body's response to allergens is to release histamine causing the mucous membranes of the nose to have which reaction? *(471)*
   1. Arterioles dilate allowing increased blood flow resulting in redness
   2. Decreased ciliary movement
   3. Rhinorrhea and watery eyes
   4. Increased surface area of the nasal passages
   5. Capillaries become more permeable causing edema and congestion

NCLEX item type: extended multiple response
Cognitive skill: recognize cues

9. The nurse recognized that the patient's symptoms in scenario #1 were probably caused by exposure to which allergens? *(Select all that apply.) (471)*
   1. Dust mites
   2. Viruses
   3. Pollens
   4. Peanuts
   5. Animal dander
   6. Feathers
   7. House dust
   8. Smoke

Copyright © 2023 by Elsevier, Inc. All rights reserved.

NCLEX item type: multiple response
Cognitive skill: explain

10. The nurse educating a patient on ways to treat rhinitis medicamentosa should provide the patient with which instructions? *(Select all that apply.)* *(472)*
    1. "The best treatment for this condition is to avoid it in the first place."
    2. "One option for you would be to work to clear one nostril at a time."
    3. "There are several treatment options available for you, but first it is important to understand the cause of the problem."
    4. "One option for you would be to completely stop taking the decongestant and work through the discomfort you will experience."
    5. "One option for you would be to switch to another decongestant—one that will not cause this condition."

NCLEX item type: multiple choice
Cognitive skill: interpret

11. A patient in scenario #1 asks the nurse what would be recommended to treat his nasal congestion from allergy symptoms. What would be an appropriate response by the nurse? *(472)*
    1. "To eliminate your symptoms, you simply must avoid the allergen."
    2. "It does not matter what type of decongestant you use, they are all very similar."
    3. "You should avoid topical decongestants as their use could cause a rebound problem that is difficult to treat."
    4. "Only use prescription medications, as the over-the-counter medications often do not work for people."

Objective: Explain the major actions (effects) of sympathomimetic, antihistaminic, and corticosteroid medicines.

NCLEX item type: multiple response
Cognitive skill: application

12. The nurse knows to watch for potential anticholinergic adverse effects of antihistamine therapy which include what symptoms? *(Select all that apply.)* *(475)*
    1. Diarrhea
    2. Stuffy nose
    3. Dry mouth
    4. Blurred vision
    5. Urinary retention

NCLEX item type: multiple choice
Cognitive skill: relate

13. The nurse explains to the patient in scenario #1 that antihistamines such as fexofenadine (Allegra) are H_1 receptor antagonists and they work by what mechanism? *(475)*
    1. Blocking the H_1 receptor sites on the target cells
    2. Causing sedation and dryness of mucous membranes
    3. Constricting the blood vessels in the nasal passages
    4. Prevent the release of histamine to reduce the symptoms of an allergic reaction

NCLEX item type: cloze
Cognitive skill: generate solutions

Choose the most likely options for the information missing from the statements below by selecting from the list of options provided.

14. The nurse explains to the patient in scenario #1 with allergic rhinitis the option to use an _____1_____ with a _____1_____ when there is inadequate response to monotherapy, and if symptoms become severe then the use of an _____2_____ and a _____2_____ and _____2_____ simultaneously may be recommended. *(472)*

Option 1	Option 2
Systemic corticosteroids	Cromolyn sodium
Antiinflammatory	Nasal corticosteroids
Decongestant	NSAIDs
Antihistamine	Antihistamine
	Decongestant

NCLEX item type: multiple choice
Cognitive skill: explain

15. Which statement does the nurse include when teaching a patient about the use of intranasal cromolyn sodium? *(478-479)*
    1. "Cromolyn sodium should not be used with a decongestant."
    2. "A 2- to 4-week course of therapy is usually required to reach full therapeutic benefit."
    3. "Cromolyn sodium should be administered as needed when symptoms occur."
    4. "Cromolyn sodium should be discontinued when the desired therapeutic response is achieved."

Copyright © 2023 by Elsevier, Inc. All rights reserved.

NCLEX item type: multiple response
Cognitive skill: application
16. Which findings does the nurse typically assess in a patient experiencing a severe allergic reaction? *(Select all that apply.)* *(471)*
    1. Dry skin
    2. Urticaria
    3. Hypertension
    4. Bronchospasms
    5. Copious secretions

Scenario #2: A patient with known hypertension and diabetes asked their healthcare provider what they should take for persistent nasal decongestion.

Objective: Explain why all decongestants products should be used cautiously by people with hypertension, hyperthyroidism, diabetes mellutis, cardiac disease, increased intraocular pressure, or prostatic disease.
NCLEX item type: multiple choice
Cognitive skill: contrast
17. When patients use nasal decongestants such as pseudoephedrine, nurses need to educate them to be aware of the possible resulting hypertension, because of which action of sympathomimetic decongestants? *(474)*
    1. Vasodilation
    2. Vasoconstriction
    3. Bronchodilation
    4. Bronchoconstriction

NCLEX item type: multiple choice
Cognitive skill: analysis
18. The patient in scenario #2 has hyperthyroidism, which prompted the nurse to caution the patient regarding the use of sympathomimetic decongestants because these agents will have what effect? *(474)*
    1. They stimulate the alpha receptors.
    2. They cause eye irritation and lacrimation.
    3. They have no effect on allergic rhinitis.
    4. They tend to produce stinging of the nasal membranes.

NCLEX item type: multiple response
Cognitive skill: application
19. The nurse consults the prescriber before administering a sympathomimetic decongestant to patients with which conditions? *(Select all that apply.)* *(474)*
    1. Glaucoma
    2. Diabetes mellitus
    3. Hypothyroidism
    4. Allergy to shellfish
    5. Prostatic hyperplasia

Objective: Discuss the nursing assessments needed during therapy to monitor the therapeutic response to and the common and serious adverse effects of decongestant drug therapy.
NCLEX item type: multiple response
Cognitive skill: take action
20. What are important premedication assessments that the nurse will include for patients who starting on decongestants? *(Select all that apply.)* *(474)*
    1. Obtain baseline vital signs
    2. Assess nasal and sinus congestion
    3. Ask about any urinary problems, especially in male patients over 55 years
    4. Review history for evidence of hypothyroidism or hypotension
    5. Determine if the patient has glaucoma or cardiac dysrhythmias and consult the healthcare provider

NCLEX item type: multiple choice
Cognitive skill: compare
21. When teaching adult patients with blocked nasal passages about the correct order to administer their intranasal corticosteroid medications, the nurse will instruct them to do what? *(477-478)*
    1. Explain that they need to administer their intranasal corticosteroid before any decongestant.
    2. Explain that they need to administer a nasal decongestant just before the intranasal therapy.
    3. Explain that they need to administer their antihistamine 30 minutes prior to the use of any decongestants.
    4. Explain that they need to avoid using a nasal decongestant; use their intranasal corticosteroid instead.

Copyright © 2023 by Elsevier, Inc. All rights reserved.

NCLEX item type: grid/matrix

Cognitive skill: recognize cues

22. The nurse reviewed the adverse effects from the medications used to treat allergic rhinitis and nasal congestion. Indicate with an 'X' which adverse effect can be see with which class of drugs. *(474,477,479)*

	Decongestants	Antihistamines	Cromolyn sodium
Blurred vision, mucosa dryness			
Bronchospasm and coughing			
Sedative effects			
Hypertension			
Urinary retention			
Nasal irritation			

Copyright © 2023 by Elsevier, Inc. All rights reserved.

Drugs Used to Treat Lower Respiratory Disease

chapter

30

Answer Key: Textbook page references are provided as a guide for answering these questions. A complete answer key is provided to your instructor.

MATCHING

Match the definition on the right with the key term on the left.

Key Term

1. _____ ventilation
2. _____ diffusion
3. _____ asthma
4. _____ bronchospasm
5. _____ goblet cells
6. _____ bronchitis

Definition

a. the movement of air in and out of the lungs
b. smooth muscle constriction causing narrowing of the airways
c. specialized mucus glands of the respiratory tract
d. a common inflammatory disease of the bronchi and bronchioles
e. a condition causing inflammation and edema with excessive mucus secretion
f. the process by which oxygen passes across the alveolar membrane to the blood

REVIEW QUESTIONS

Scenario #1: A 75-year-old male patient was admitted to the hospital with respiratory failure secondary to pneumonia. After several days of being treated with steroids and antibiotics, he has stabilized on 2 L of oxygen via nasal cannula. He has a history of chronic obstructive pulmonary disease (COPD), congestive heart failure, hypothyroidism, and rheumatoid arthritis, all of which are currently medically managed.

Objective: Discuss nursing assessments used to evaluate the respiratory status of a patient.

NCLEX item type: multiple choice
Cognitive skill: take action

7. A nurse is assessing the patient in scenario #1 and listens to lung sounds. Which findings would the nurse report to the healthcare provider for further evaluation? *(484,490)*
   1. Elevated shoulders and use of abdominal muscles to breathe
   2. Dry nonproductive cough
   3. Coughing up thin, white secretions
   4. Rapid, shallow breathing with O_2 saturation of 88%

NCLEX item type: multiple response
Cognitive skill: application

8. During a respiratory assessment of the patient in scenario #1, the nurse listens to breath sounds and monitors the respiratory rate, as well as what other symptoms? *(Select all that apply.)* *(490)*
   1. Appetite
   2. Mental status
   3. Urine output
   4. Signs of cyanosis
   5. Use of abdominal muscles during breathing

NCLEX item type: multiple response
Cognitive skill: interpret

9. The nurse will check which laboratory and diagnostic tests in order to understand the patient's diagnosis? *(Select all that apply.)* *(490)*
   1. ABGs
   2. Chest X-rays
   3. Creatinine clearance
   4. Electrocardiograph
   5. Pulmonary function tests

Copyright © 2023 by Elsevier, Inc. All rights reserved.

NCLEX item type: multiple response
Cognitive skill: explain

10. The nurse needs to educate patients who have respiratory conditions on important health maintenance aspects, which include what instructions? *(Select all that apply.)* *(491)*
    1. Hand hygiene to prevent infections
    2. Encourage an increase in fluid intake
    3. Follow prescribed medications when feeling short of breath
    4. Humidify the air to relieve dryness
    5. Use of abdominal muscles during breathing

NCLEX item type: multiple choice
Cognitive skill: relate

11. The nurse was discussing the timing of the administration of medications for the patient in scenario #2 with asthma. Which statement by the nurse is correct? *(492)*
    1. "It does not matter in which order you take your medications."
    2. "Take your steroid inhaler first, then your bronchodilator."
    3. "Take your bronchodilator first, then your steroid inhaler."
    4. "Take your bronchodilator first, then wait 2 hours before taking your steroid inhaler."

NCLEX item type: multiple choice
Cognitive skill: evaluate

12. The nurse is explaining the different zones of a peak flowmeter to the patient with asthma and how to use it to assess when symptoms are changing. The nurse recognizes that the patient needs further teaching after the patient in scenario #2 makes which statement? *(491)*
    1. "The green zone is good, the yellow zone is warning, and the red zone is danger."
    2. "I can use the quick-relief medication when I notice that I am in the yellow zone."
    3. "The quick-relief medication and corticosteroids are used when I am in the green zone."
    4. "The peak flowmeter measures my peak expiratory flow and helps me determine how to manage my asthma."

Objective: Distinguish the mechanisms of action of expectorants, antitussives, and mucolytic agents.

NCLEX item type: multiple choice
Cognitive skill: compare

13. The nurse expects that an effective cough suppressant and the standard against which other antitussive agents are compared is which medication? *(493)*
    1. codeine
    2. guaifenesin
    3. ipratropium
    4. acetylcysteine

NCLEX item type: multiple choice
Cognitive skill: classify

14. The nurse explains to the patient in scenario #1 that expectorants are those drugs whose action is to do what? *(493)*
    1. Relax the smooth muscles of the airway.
    2. Suppress the cough center in the brain.
    3. Increase the viscosity of mucus plugs.
    4. Enhance the flow of respiratory secretions, which promotes ciliary action.

NCLEX item type: multiple choice
Cognitive skill: explain

15. The nurse was educating the patient on what to expect from mucolytics, and described them as having what action? *(495)*
    1. "These agents play an important role in the treatment of asthma to reduce inflammation."
    2. "These agents relax the smooth muscle of the tracheobronchial tree."
    3. "These agents inhibit a key enzyme from being metabolizes allowing it to accumulate and reduce inflammation."
    4. "These agents reduce the stickiness and viscosity of pulmonary secretions by acting directly on the mucus plugs to dissolve them."

NCLEX item type: multiple response
Cognitive skill: application

16. The nurse gives which instructions to a patient prior to the administration of an antitussive agent? *(Select all that apply.)* *(494)*
    1. "Be sure to drink plenty of liquids to keep hydrated."
    2. "Remember, this drug may cause you to become sleepy."
    3. "You need to describe the characteristics of your cough."
    4. "It would be wise to record your peak expiratory flow prior to use."
    5. "You need to make sure you have your nebulizing equipment for administration."

NCLEX item type: multiple choice
Cognitive skill: compare

17. When administering guaifenesin to a patient with bronchitis, the nurse expects that the drug will have what effect? *(493)*
    1. Dilate the bronchioles
    2. Thin the bronchial secretions
    3. Increase the viscosity of mucus secretions
    4. Increase the frequency of a nonproductive cough

Copyright © 2023 by Elsevier, Inc. All rights reserved.

NCLEX item type: multiple choice
Cognitive skill: interpret
18. The nurse will assess the action of acetylcysteine as working when the patient exhibits which symptom? *(495)*
    1. Kussmaul's respiration
    2. Increased nonproductive coughing
    3. Thicker and more viscous secretions
    4. Improved airway flow and more comfortable breathing

Objective: Describe the nursing assessments needed to monitor therapeutic response and the development of adverse effects from beta-adrenergic bronchodilator therapy.
NCLEX item type: multiple choice
Cognitive skill: comprehension
19. The nurse will observe for an expected effect from beta-adrenergic agents on patients with respiratory conditions such as asthma. Which effect will be expected from beta-adrenergic agents? *(495-496)*
    1. Bronchodilation causing easier breathing
    2. Increase in respiratory rate
    3. Thinner respiratory secretions
    4. Decrease in peak expiratory flow
NCLEX item type: extended multiple choice
Cognitive skill: recognize cues
20. The patient in scenario #2 is given beta-adrenergic agents, and the nurse needs to monitor for which systemic adverse effects? *(Select all that apply.)* *(497)*
    1. Nausea, vomiting
    2. Sedation
    3. Urinary retention
    4. Palpitations
    5. Restlessness
    6. Nervousness
    7. Cardiac arrhythmias
    8. Lethargy
    9. Anxiety
    10. Tachycardia
NCLEX item type: multiple response
Cognitive skill: compare
21. The nurse recognized the short-acting beta-adrenergic agents that have a rapid onset and are used to treat acute bronchospasms as these drugs. Which medications are included in this drug class? *(Select all that apply.)* *(496)*
    1. albuterol
    2. dipropionate
    3. salmeterol
    4. tiotropium

    5. levalbuterol
NCLEX item type: cloze
Cognitive skill: recognize cues
Choose the most likely options for the information missing from the statements below by selecting from the list of options provided.
22. The nurse expects that _____1_____drugs will enhance the effect of beta-adrenergic bronchodilators and inhibit_____2_____ responses that may result in ____3_____. *(499)*

Option 1	Option 2	Option 3
Antileukotriene agents		Cough reflex
Corticosteroid inhalants	Allergic	Bronchocon-striction
Anticholinergic bronchodilators	Inflammatory	Increased secretions
Phosphdiesterase-4 inhibitors		Cyanosis

Scenario #2: A 35-year-old patient diagnosed with asthma came to the clinic to have a checkup and medication adjustment. The patient asks the nurse to explain some of the bronchodilators that were prescribed and why they needed them.

Objective: Discuss the nursing assessments needed to monitor therapeutic response and the development of adverse effects from anticholinergic bronchodilator therapy.
NCLEX item type: multiple choice
Cognitive skill: illustrate
23. The nurse reviewed the expected actions of the anticholinergic bronchodilator agents that the patient in scenario #2 was on for treatment asthma. Which effect is the expected outcome for these drugs? *(499)*
    1. They inhibit the inflammatory response in the bronchioles.
    2. They stabilize the mast cells to prevent the release of histamine.
    3. They block the cholinergic effect of bronchial constriction by the vagus nerve.
    4. They bind to the circulating antibodies in the blood, making them not as available to trigger symptoms.

Copyright © 2023 by Elsevier, Inc. All rights reserved.

NCLEX item type: multiple response
Cognitive skill: application
24. The nurse knows anticholinergic agents have potent adverse effects that limit their use. Which effects are important to monitor the patient for who is taking anticholinergic agents? *(Select all that apply.) (499)*
    1. Mydriasis
    2. Bradycardia
    3. Tachycardia
    4. Urinary retention
    5. Throat irritation

NCLEX item type: multiple choice
Cognitive skill: contrast
25. The nurse reviewed the medications prescribed for the patient in scenario #1. Which ones are used to treat COPD? *(Select all that apply.) (498,500)*
    1. tiotropium (Spiriva)
    2. spironolactone (Aldactone)
    3. levothyroxine (Synthroid)
    4. indomethacin (Indocin)
    5. budesonide (Pulmicort)

Objective: Discuss the nursing assessments needed to monitor therapeutic response and the development of adverse effects from corticosteroid inhalant therapy.

NCLEX item type: multiple response
Cognitive skill: application
26. The nurse will assess the important components of blood gases that indicate overall pulmonary function. Which values are needed to be monitored? *(Select all that apply.) (484)*
    1. Pao_2
    2. pH
    3. $Paco_2$
    4. HCO_3
    5. Hgb

NCLEX item type: multiple choice
Cognitive skill: contrast
27. Which component of blood gases measures the ratio of actual oxygen content of hemoglobin compared with the hemoglobin's ability to carry oxygen? *(484)*
    1. Sao_2
    2. Pao_2
    3. pH
    4. $Paco_2$

NCLEX item type: multiple response
Cognitive skill: application
28. What instructions will the nurse give the patient in scenario #2 who is started on systemic steroids for exacerbation of asthma? *(499-501)*
    1. "Your corticosteroid inhalant therapy will be discontinued while you take these steroids orally."
    2. "Your bronchodilator inhalant agents will be discontinued while you take these steroids orally."
    3. "These steroids are given to allow easier breathing with less effort by decreasing pulmonary inflammation."
    4. "The full therapeutic benefit from these systemic steroids may require up to 4 weeks of therapy for maximum benefit."
    5. "It is important to remember that oral thrush can develop with inhaled steroids as well as large oral doses of corticosteroids, be sure to gargle and rinse the mouth after treatment."

Copyright © 2023 by Elsevier, Inc. All rights reserved.

Drugs Used to Treat Oral Disorders

chapter

31

Answer Key: Textbook page references are provided as a guide for answering these questions. A complete answer key is provided to your instructor.

MATCHING
Match the definition on the right with the key term on the left.

Key Term

1. _____ canker sores
2. _____ candidiasis
3. _____ plaque
4. _____ gingivitis
5. _____ halitosis
6. _____ xerostomia
7. _____ mucositis

Definition

a. a painful inflammation of the mucous membranes of the mouth
b. an oral fungal infection
c. a condition in which the flow of saliva is decreased or completely stopped
d. oral lesions usually gray to whitish-yellow with a red halo of inflamed tissue
e. a whitish-yellow substance that builds up on teeth and gum lines
f. foul mouth odor
g. inflammation of the gums

REVIEW QUESTIONS

Scenario #1: A 52-year-old female patient arrives at the outpatient clinic with complaints of painful mouth lesions around her lower gums. The patient was diagnosed with canker sores and treatment was started to control the pain and facilitate healing.

Objectives: Explain common oral disorders and their treatments.
NCLEX item type: multiple choice
Cognitive skill: explain

8. The patient in scenario #1 asks the nurse in the clinic what could have been done to prevent these painful sores from developing. Which statement would be appropriate for the nurse to say? *(508-509)*
   1. "Everybody gets them, they will go away eventually; I would not worry about it."
   2. "Proper oral hygiene, such as brushing your teeth after eating, will prevent them."
   3. "You probably should have seen a dentist twice a year to prevent them."
   4. "The exact cause is unknown, but stress and trauma are precipitating factors."

NCLEX item type: multiple choice
Cognitive skill: knowledge

9. The nurse discussed with the patient who had xerostomia the treatment options available. Which statement by the nurse is correct? *(510)*
   1. "You can use mouthwashes to freshen the breath."
   2. "You can use a saliva substitute for this condition."
   3. "You can use topical analgesics to reduce the pain."
   4. "You can use an oral irrigation and proper oral hygiene."

NCLEX item type: multiple response
Cognitive skill: application

10. Patients who are being treated for cold sores should be taught by the nurse to use which treatment option? *(Select all that apply.) (510)*
    1. Purchase docosanol (Abreva) over the counter to treat the cold sore
    2. Keep the mouth moist to prevent cracking and prevent secondary infection
    3. Gently wash the cold sore with soap and water
    4. Use topical antibiotic ointment such as Neosporin as soon as lesions occur
    5. Use topical analgesics and sun protection products

Copyright © 2023 by Elsevier, Inc. All rights reserved.

NCLEX item type: cloze
Cognitive skill: recognize cues

Choose the most likely options for the information missing from the statements below by selecting from the list of options provided.

11. The common mouth disorder _____1_____ can be seen in _____2_____, _____2_____, and _____2_____ and is characterized by white milk-curd–appearing plaques attached to the oral mucosa. *(509)*

Option 1	Option 2
Mucositis	Debilitated patients
Gingivitis	Infants
Candidiasis	Athletes
Xerostomia	Pregnant women

NCLEX item type: multiple response
Cognitive skill: generate solutions

12. When discussing ways to prevent or treat halitosis, the nurse explains to a patient which measures to take? *(Select all that apply.) (509-510)*
    1. Flossing regularly
    2. Using mouthwashes
    3. Brushing at least twice a day
    4. Applying Vaseline to the lips
    5. Taking antifungal medications

NCLEX item type: multiple choice
Cognitive skill: knowledge

13. The nurse discusses the proper oral hygiene of brushing twice a day to patients in order to prevent what oral disorder? *(509)*
    1. Sinusitis
    2. Xerostomia
    3. Plaque
    4. Canker sores

NCLEX item type: multiple choice
Cognitive skill: compare

14. The nurse caring for a patient undergoing chemotherapy reminds the patient that effective oral care with alcohol-free mouth rinses and frequent tooth brushing will help prevent which oral disorder? *(511)*
    1. Canker sores
    2. Xerostomia
    3. Mucositis
    4. Cold sores

Objective: Identify nursing assessments and interventions associated with the treatment of mucositis.

NCLEX item type: multiple response
Cognitive skill: application

15. Nurses need to perform an oral assessment in patients susceptible to mouth disorders to detect any abnormal findings such as what? *(Select all that apply.) (511)*
    1. Well-fitting dentures
    2. Red, swollen gum line
    3. Pink, moist mucous membranes
    4. White patches over the tongue
    5. Teeth coated with food particles

NCLEX item type: multiple response
Cognitive skill: application

16. Which action will the nurse teach the patient as an effective treatment for relief of symptoms caused by mucositis? *(Select all that apply.) (511)*
    1. Rinsing the mouth before and after meals
    2. Viscous lidocaine 2% can be used before meals to relieve pain
    3. Using commercially prepared mouthwash with alcohol
    4. Mucosal protectants such as Gelcair or Orabase work by coating the mucosa
    5. Nystatin liquid suspension swished and swallowed

Copyright © 2023 by Elsevier, Inc. All rights reserved.

Drugs Used to Treat Gastroesophageal Reflux and Peptic Ulcer Diseases

chapter

32

Answer Key: Textbook page references are provided as a guide for answering these questions. A complete answer key is provided to your instructor.

MATCHING
Match the definition on the right with the key term on the left.

Key Term

1. _____ gastroesophageal reflux disease (GERD)
2. _____ peptic ulcer disease (PUD)
3. _____ *Helicobacter pylori*
4. _____ heartburn
5. _____ mucus cells
6. _____ parietal cells
7. _____ chief cells
8. _____ hydrochloric acid

Definition

a. secretory cells of the stomach that secrete hydrochloric acid
b. acid indigestion
c. secretory cells of the stomach that secrete pepsinogen
d. symptoms include epigastric pain noted when the stomach is empty
e. bacteria that are able to live below the mucus barrier of the stomach
f. the reflux of gastric secretions up into the esophagus
g. activates pepsinogen to pepsin providing the optimal pH
h. secretory cells of the stomach that secrete mucus

REVIEW QUESTIONS

Scenario #1: A 38-year-old male patient came into the clinic with complaints of acid indigestion and reflux and was diagnosed with GERD and prescribed an H$_2$ receptor antagonist and an antacid.

Objective: Discuss common stomach disorders that require drug therapy.
NCLEX item type: multiple response
Cognitive skill: application
9. The nurse assured the patient in scenario #1 that they had been prescribed an appropriate treatment for their GERD, in addition they could have been prescribed agents from which class of drugs? *(Select all that apply.)* **(519)**
   1. Coating agents
   2. Proton pump inhibitors
   3. Prokinetic agents
   4. Nonsteroidal antiinflammatory drugs
   5. Beta-adrenergic blocking agents

NCLEX item type: multiple response
Cognitive skill: compare
10. Which of these stomach disorders are treated with proton pump inhibitors? *(Select all that apply.)* **(525)**
    1. GERD
    2. Severe esophagitis
    3. Zollinger-Ellison syndrome
    4. Hiatal hernia
    5. Peptic ulcer disease

NCLEX item type: multiple choice
Cognitive skill: knowledge
11. The nurse reviewed the drug used for patients with gastroparesis, which stimulate gastric emptying and increases intestinal transit. Which drug is a gastric stimulant as well as an antiemetic? **(527)**
    1. cimetidine
    2. omeprazole
    3. sucralfate
    4. metoclopramide

Scenario #2: A patient admitted to the hospital with GI bleeding had been vomiting blood and confirmed having severe abdominal pain for several weeks prior to this episode. The patient was diagnosed with a gastric ulcer and started on proper treatment.

Copyright © 2023 by Elsevier, Inc. All rights reserved.

Objective: Identify factors that prevent breakdown of the body's normal defense barriers resulting in ulcer formation.

NCLEX item type: multiple choice
Cognitive skill: classify

12. The nurse explained to the patient in scenario #2 that one of the known causes of peptic ulcer disease is an infection in the mucosal wall of the stomach caused by an organism. Which organism will the nurse discuss? *(518)*
    1. *Escherichia coli*
    2. *Helicobacter pylori*
    3. *Streptococcus viridans*
    4. *Staphylococcus aureus*

NCLEX item type: multiple response
Cognitive skill: application

13. The nurse understands that patients older than 65 years with ulcer disease usually present with which symptoms? *(Select all that apply.)* *(521)*
    1. Weight loss
    2. Anorexia
    3. Dizziness
    4. Vague abdominal discomfort
    5. Burning in the epigastric region

NCLEX item type: multiple response
Cognitive skill: application

14. The nurse discussed the risk factors that increase the likelihood of developing peptic ulcer disease with the patient in scenario #2. Which factors did the nurse discuss? *(Select all that apply.)* *(518)*
    1. Cigarette smoking
    2. Spicy foods and alcohol
    3. An infection in the stomach lining
    4. An increase in stress level
    5. Injury to the mucosal lining of the stomach by NSAIDs

Objective: Discuss the drug classifications and actions used to treat stomach disorders.

NCLEX item type: cloze
Cognitive skill: recognize cues

Choose the most likely options for the information missing from the statements below by selecting from the list of options provided.

15. The nurse knows that _____ a class of medication used in the treatment of peptic ulcer will inhibit gastric secretion of hydrochloric acid by inhibiting the hydrogen ion pump of the _____ cells? *(522)*

Option 1	Option 2
Proton pump inhibitors	Chief
Histamine receptor antagonists	Mucous
Coating agents	Parietal
Antacids	Mast

NCLEX item type: multiple choice
Cognitive skill: compare

16. The nurse recognized the agents used in the treatment of GERD and PUD and for preventing gastric ulcers in critically ill patients by causing the pH of the stomach to rise are which class? *(520)*
    1. Antacids
    2. Coating agents
    3. Gastrointestinal prostaglandin
    4. Histamine-2 receptor antagonists

Objective: Identify interventions that incorporate pharmacologic and nonpharmacologic treatments for an individual with stomach disorders.

NCLEX item type: multiple choice
Cognitive skill: analyze

17. Which statement does the nurse include when teaching the patient in scenario #2 about antacid therapy for the treatment of peptic ulcer disease? *(521)*
    1. "Antacids take at least 6 weeks to become effective."
    2. "Excessive use of magnesium antacids results in constipation."
    3. "Antacid tablets do not contain enough antacid to be effective in treating this disease."
    4. "A common complaint of patients using large quantities of calcium carbonate antacids is diarrhea."

NCLEX item type: multiple choice
Cognitive skill: knowledge

18. A patient with a history of chronic renal failure is on high-dose cimetidine (Tagamet HB) therapy for the treatment of a duodenal ulcer. It is most important for the nurse to assess the patient for which adverse effect of this therapy? *(523)*
    1. Diarrhea
    2. Dizziness
    3. Constipation
    4. Disorientation

NCLEX item type: multiple response
Cognitive skill: application

19. The nurse was teaching the patient in scenario #1 about the use of antacids as part of the treatment for GERD. Which statements by the nurse will be included in the discussion? *(Select all that apply.)* *(521)*
    1. "Maalox is an example of a low-sodium antacid."
    2. "Use of an antacid with large amounts of magnesium usually results in constipation."
    3. "Calcium carbonate and sodium bicarbonate may cause rebound hyperacidity."
    4. "Patients with renal failure should not use large quantities of antacids containing magnesium."
    5. "Antacid tablets should be used only for patients with occasional indigestion or heartburn."

Copyright © 2023 by Elsevier, Inc. All rights reserved.

NCLEX item type: multiple response
Cognitive skill: evaluate outcomes
20. The nurse reviewed the uses for the different drug classes used to treat common gastric disorders. *(520,524,526,527)*

Mark with an 'arrow' the drug class used for the gastric disorder. Mark each drug class only once, indicating the most common use.

Drug Class	Gastric disorder
Prokinetic agents	Gastric ulcers
Antacids	GERD
Proton pump inhibitors	Indigestion
Coating agents	Gastroparesis

Copyright © 2023 by Elsevier, Inc. All rights reserved.

Drugs Used to Treat Nausea and Vomiting

Answer Key: Textbook page references are provided as a guide for answering these questions. A complete answer key is provided to your instructor.

MATCHING
Match the key terms on the left with the definitions on the right.

Key Terms

1. _____ emetogenicity
2. _____ psychogenic vomiting
3. _____ regurgitation
4. _____ hyperemesis gravidarum
5. _____ delayed emesis
6. _____ radiation-induced nausea and vomiting (RINV)
7. _____ chemotherapy-induced nausea and vomiting (CINV)

Definitions

a. a common cause of emesis associated with the treatment of cancer
b. a condition in which starvation, dehydration, and acidosis are superimposed on the vomiting syndrome
c. having the ability to cause emesis
d. the most unpleasant adverse effect from chemotherapy
e. when the gastric or esophageal contents rise to the pharynx because of greater pressure in the stomach
f. usually starts more than 24 hours after chemotherapy treatment ends
g. chronic or recurrent vomiting that can be self-induced or occur involuntarily in response to threatening or distasteful situations

REVIEW QUESTIONS

Scenario #1: A 26-year-old pregnant woman came to the outpatient clinic complaining about severe persistent vomiting for the past several weeks. She states that it is impossible to keep anything down and now she is getting weak.

Objective: Describe the common causes of nausea and vomiting and the interventions that apply.
NCLEX item type: multiple choice
Cognitive skill: knowledge

8. The nurse recognized that nausea and vomiting symptoms associated with motion sickness are thought to result from stimulation of what? *(532)*
   1. The diaphragm
   2. The cerebral cortex
   3. The labyrinth system of the ear
   4. The sensory receptors on the tongue and soft palate

NCLEX item type: extended multiple choice
Cognitive skill: recognize cues

9. The nurse knows there are six common causes of nausea and vomiting. Which ones will the nurse recognize? *(Select all that apply.) (532-534)*
   1. motion sickness
   2. nausea and vomiting in pregnancy
   3. delayed emesis
   4. chemotherapy-induced nausea and vomiting
   5. anticipatory nausea and vomiting
   6. radiation-induced nausea and vomiting
   7. psychogenic vomiting
   8. postoperative nausea and vomiting

Copyright © 2023 by Elsevier, Inc. All rights reserved.

NCLEX item type: multiple choice
Cognitive skill: classify
10. The patient in scenario #1 has which condition in which starvation, dehydration, and acidosis are superimposed on the vomiting, requiring hospitalization? *(533)*
    1. Drug toxicity
    2. Regurgitation
    3. Delayed emesis
    4. Hyperemesis gravidarum

NCLEX item type: multiple response
Cognitive skill: application
11. Patients who have cancer and are undergoing treatment with gamma rays and chemotherapy may develop the adverse effect of nausea and vomiting, which is called what? *(Select all that apply.)* *(533-534)*
    1. Delayed emesis
    2. Psychogenic vomiting
    3. CINV
    4. PONV
    5. RINV

NCLEX item type: multiple choice
Cognitive skill: interpret
12. The nurse is educating a patient prescribed diphenhydramine (Benadryl) for motion sickness, and knows the patient needs more teaching after hearing which response? *(539)*
    1. "I understand that I should not drive a car after taking this."
    2. "This drug has fewer side effects than promethazine."
    3. "I will call my provider if I notice that I am starting to have trouble urinating."
    4. "I have taken this before so I know that my mouth gets really dry, and for that I have some candy to suck on."

NCLEX item type: multiple choice
Cognitive skill: comprehension
13. The nurse understands that antiemetic agents be administered to be considered most effective when given at what time? *(534)*
    1. It does not matter
    2. Before the onset of nausea
    3. After nausea has occurred
    4. After vomiting has occurred

Scenario #2: A patient undergoing chemotherapy for treatment of lung cancer came into the outpatient department for treatment after having a long-term catheter inserted for this purpose.

Objective: Discuss the three types of nausea associated with chemotherapy and the nursing considerations.
NCLEX item type: cloze
Cognitive skill: recognize cues
Choose the most likely options for the information missing from the statements below by selecting from the list of options provided.
14. The nurse explains to the patient in scenario #2 that _____1_____ and _____1_____ are therapies used for cancer treatment. Adverse effects from these treatments can cause nausea and vomiting and the three type associated with chemotherapy are _____2____, ____2_____, and _____2_____. *(533-534)*

Option 1	Option 2
Chemotherapy	Hyperemesis gravidarum
Medication therapy	Anticipatory nausea and vomiting
Hyperbaric chamber	Delayed emesis
Radiation therapy	Regurgitation
Relaxation therapy	Acute nausea and vomiting

NCLEX item type: multiple response
Cognitive skill: application
15. What are the various ways that the nurse can teach the patient in scenario #2 about the treatment of chemotherapy induced nausea and vomiting with antiemetics? *(Select all that apply.)* *(535)*
    1. Patients are given a combination of antiemetic agents.
    2. Patients are given emetogenic agents to prevent delayed emesis.
    3. Patients are administered antiemetics prior to chemotherapy.
    4. Patients are encouraged to use over-the-counter herbal supplements for treatment.
    5. Patients are to continue antiemetic therapy for several weeks following chemotherapy.

NCLEX item type: multiple response
Cognitive skill: contrast
16. The nurse can expect that the patient in scenario #2 starting on the antineoplastic agent cisplatin will need to take a combination of antiemetics. Which two agents work best for highly emetogenic anticancer agents? *(Select all that apply.)* *(535)*
    1. metoclopramide
    2. dexamethasone
    3. amisulpride
    4. diphenhydramine
    5. dronabinol

Copyright © 2023 by Elsevier, Inc. All rights reserved.

NCLEX item type: multiple response
Cognitive skill: application
17. The nurse explained to the patient who recently underwent radiation therapy about which factors that influence RINV? *(Select all that apply.)* **(534)**
    1. The treatment site
    2. The total dose delivered
    3. The dose of radiation delivered
    4. The number of cancer cells radiated
    5. The previous development of nausea and vomiting

Objective: Compare the therapeutic classes of antiemetics with their uses.
NCLEX item type: multiple choice
Cognitive skill: explain
18. The nurse was talking with a patient who mentioned they heard that marijuana is used for nausea now and would like some for their symptoms. What would be the best response by the nurse? **(547)**
    1. "You cannot have any marijuana. It is illegal."
    2. "I will have to ask your doctor if it would be okay for you to have any."
    3. "I heard it does not really help patients who are nauseated. I would not recommend it."
    4. "The active ingredient in marijuana has been made into a medication that your doctor may prescribe for you."

NCLEX item type: multiple choice
Cognitive skill: compare
19. The nurse explains to the patient that most antiemetic agents used to reduce nausea and vomiting from motion sickness are chemically related to what drug class? **(534)**
    1. Antiepileptics
    2. Analgesics
    3. Antihistamines
    4. Anticoagulants

NCLEX item type: multiple response
Cognitive skill: classify
20. The nurse was considering the antiemetic medications available and understands that certain ones would be of benefit to give to the patient in scenario #2. Which options are available for control of nausea and vomiting with chemotherapy? *(Select all that apply.)* **(535)**
    1. Benzodiazepines (e.g., lorazepam, diazepam)
    2. Corticosteroids (e.g., dexamethasone)
    3. Antihistamines (e.g., diphenhydramine, meclizine)
    4. Neurokinin-1 antagonists (e.g., aprepitant, fosaprepitant)
    5. Serotonin antagonists (e.g., ondansetron)

Copyright © 2023 by Elsevier, Inc. All rights reserved.

Drugs Used to Treat Constipation and Diarrhea

Answer Key: Textbook page references are provided as a guide for answering these questions. A complete answer key is provided to your instructor.

MATCHING
Match the drug class on the left with the action of the drugs on the right.

Drug Class

1. _____ stimulant laxatives
2. _____ osmotic laxatives
3. _____ saline laxatives
4. _____ lubricant laxatives
5. _____ bulk-forming laxatives
6. _____ stool softeners
7. _____ peripheral opioid antagonists

Drug Action

a. bind to opioid receptors in the GI tract, inhibiting the constipating effects of opioids
b. lubricate the intestinal wall and soften the stool
c. cause water to be retained within the stool and increases bulk, which stimulates peristalsis
d. cause an irritation of the intestine that promotes peristalsis and evacuation
e. magnesium-containing products that stimulate muscle peristalsis to aid in evacuation
f. hypertonic compounds that draw water into the intestine from surrounding tissues
g. wetting agents that draw water into the stool, causing it to soften

REVIEW QUESTIONS
Scenario #1: A patient who is seeing their healthcare provider for a follow-up after surgery came to the clinic and during the interview and assessment by the nurse mentioned the problem of constipation they had been experiencing since taking pain medication.

Objective: Identify the mechanism of action for the different classes of laxatives, and describe underlying causes of constipation.
NCLEX item type: multiple response
Cognitive skill: application

8. A patient asked the nurse for some advice on how to prevent constipation that was bothering them lately. Which response by the nurse would be appropriate? *(Select all that apply.)* **(551)**
   1. "Do you have any history of diseases of the stomach?"
   2. "What type of diet do you follow? One with plenty of fruits and vegetables should help."
   3. "Tell me about your daily activity level. Being physically active helps eliminate problems."
   4. "Have you ever been told you have anemia or hypothyroidism? These conditions predispose you to constipation."
   5. "Tell me about the medications you are taking. Certain types of drugs can cause constipation."

NCLEX item type: multiple choice
Cognitive skill: compare

9. The nurse reviewed the mechanism of action of stimulant laxatives. Which action do these laxative have? **(554)**
   1. They draw water into the stool, causing it to soften.
   2. They add lubrication to the intestinal wall and soften the stool.
   3. They draw water into the intestine from surrounding tissues by means of hypertonic compounds.
   4. They act directly on the intestine, causing irritation that promotes peristalsis and evacuation.

NCLEX item type: multiple choice
Cognitive skill: explain

10. Which statement does the nurse include when teaching a patient about the use of osmotic laxatives? **(554)**
    1. "These agents usually work within 8–12 hours."
    2. "Osmotic laxatives restore normal intestinal flora."
    3. "Osmotic laxatives work by making the stool softer."
    4. "Glycerin suppositories usually act within 15 to 30 minutes."

Copyright © 2023 by Elsevier, Inc. All rights reserved.

NCLEX item type: multiple choice
Cognitive skill: illustrate
11. The patient asks the nurse how mineral oil works as a laxative. What statement by the nurse explains the mechanism of action of lubricant laxatives? *(555)*
    1. "The lubricant laxatives are used because they increase peristalsis."
    2. "Mineral oil will work by drawing more water into the stool."
    3. "Lubricant laxatives work by increasing bulk in the stool to stimulate peristalsis."
    4. "Mineral oil will lubricate the intestinal wall and soften the stool to allow a smooth passage of fecal contents."

NCLEX item type: multiple choice
Cognitive skill: application
12. The nurse was explaining how bulk-forming laxatives work to the patient who had a recent order for psyllium. Which statement by the nurse need to be corrected? *(Select all that apply.)* *(555)*
    1. "Bulk-forming laxatives are used to relieve acute constipation."
    2. "Bulk-forming laxatives are used to treat certain types of diarrhea."
    3. "Adequate volumes of water must be taken with bulk-forming laxatives, such as psyllium."
    4. "Bulk-forming laxatives may be used in the treatment of patients with irritable bowel syndrome."
    5. "The drug of choice for people who are incapacitated and need a laxative regularly are the bulk-forming laxatives."

NCLEX item type: multiple choice
Cognitive skill: knowledge
13. The nurse was teaching the patient in scenario #1 that a stool softener helps to prevent constipation from pain medications. What is the mechanism of action of stool softeners that the nurse taught the patient? *(555)*
    1. Stool softeners lubricate the intestines.
    2. Stool softeners stimulate peristalsis.
    3. Stool softeners add bulk to the stool.
    4. Stool softeners draw water into the stool, causing it to soften.

Scenario #2: A 72-year-old patient admitted to the hospital with recent mental status changes, gastroesophageal reflux disease (GERD), and symptoms of gastric outlet obstruction was being managed with a nasogastric (NG) tube. The patient has a history of Crohn disease with a bowel resection resulting in an ileostomy and was experiencing high output from the ileostomy.

Objective: Discuss the causes of diarrhea.
NCLEX item type: multiple response
Cognitive skill: application
14. The nurse knows there are conditions that predispose patients to developing diarrhea. Which conditions would apply to this development? *(Select all that apply.)* *(552)*
    1. Anemia
    2. Hypothyroidism
    3. Crohn disease
    4. Hyperthyroidism
    5. Enzyme deficiencies

NCLEX item type: multiple response
Cognitive skill: illustrate
15. Diet is an important consideration for patients who have developed diarrhea. The nurse educates the patient on which food items to avoid to prevent diarrhea? *(Select all that apply.)* *(552)*
    1. Spicy foods
    2. Fresh oysters
    3. Deep-fat fried foods
    4. Cheese and yogurt
    5. Drinking tap water when on vacation in another country

NCLEX item type: multiple choice
Cognitive skill: knowledge
16. The nurse recognized the condition that the patient in scenario #2 has that is an example of a common cause of diarrhea. Which condition is likely responsible for the diarrhea? *(552)*
    1. GERD
    2. Crohn disease
    3. Mental status changes
    4. Gastric outlet obstruction

Objective: Differentiate between locally acting and systemically acting antidiarrheal agents and the conditions that respond favorably to antidiarrheal agents.
NCLEX item type: multiple response
Cognitive skill: application
17. The nurse recognized the mechanism of action of loperamide (Imodium) a systemically acting antidiarrheal agent. Which action does this drug have on the patient? *(Select all that apply.)* *(558)*
    1. Imodium will promote the expulsion of formed stool.
    2. Imodium will absorb nutrients, water, and electrolytes and leave a formed stool.
    3. Imodium increases peristalsis and GI motility via the autonomic nervous system.
    4. Imodium decreases peristalsis and GI motility via the autonomic nervous system.
    5. Imodium draws water from the surrounding tissues into the GI tract.

Copyright © 2023 by Elsevier, Inc. All rights reserved.

NCLEX item type: cloze
Cognitive skill: recognize cues

Choose the most likely options for the information missing from the statements below by selecting from the list of options provided.

18. The nurse was administering _____1_____ a locally acting antidiarrheal agent, and knows it works by the mechanism of actions that _____2_____and _____2_____.
(558)

Option 1	Option 2
bismuth subsalicylate (Pepto-Bismol)	Slow the motility of the GI tract
diphenoxylate with atropine (Lomotil)	Absorbs excess water to cause a formed stool
lubiprostone (Amitiza)	Irritate the lining of the GI tract
docusate sodium (Colace)	Absorbs irritants or bacteria that are causing diarrhea

Objective: Describe nursing assessments needed to evaluate the patient's state of hydration when suffering from either constipation or dehydration, and identify electrolytes that should be monitored whenever prolonged or severe diarrhea is present.

NCLEX item type: multiple response
Cognitive skill: application

19. The nurse will need to monitor which laboratory values that may indicate a problem with malabsorption or dehydration for the patient in scenario #2? *(Select all that apply.)* *(553)*
    1. Chloride
    2. Potassium
    3. Bicarbonate
    4. Blood sugar
    5. Alkaline phosphate

NCLEX item type: multiple response
Cognitive skill: recognize cues

20. Assessments of the patient in scenario #2 made by the nurse to determine if dehydration is present include checking which factors? *(Select all that apply.)* *(553)*
    1. Weight loss
    2. Excessive appetite
    3. Inelastic skin turgor
    4. Poor urine output
    5. Sticky mucous membranes

NCLEX item type: multiple choice
Cognitive skill: compare

21. The patient in the scenario experiencing increased ileostomy output would likely receive which drug to inhibit peristalsis and reduce the volume from the ileostomy? *(558)*
    1. lactulose (Constulose)
    2. diphenoxylate with atropine (Lomotil)
    3. bisacodyl (Dulcolax)
    4. naldemedine (Symproic)

NCLEX item type: grid/matrix
Cognitive skill: analyze cues

22. The nurse reviewed the conditions that cause constipation and diarrhea. Indicate with an 'X' which patient condition causes which GI symptom. *(551-552)*

	Constipation	Diarrhea
Anemia		
paraplegic		
Tumors of the bowel		
Colitis		
Crohn disease		
Small bowel obstruction		
GI surgery		
Inflammatory bowel disease		

Copyright © 2023 by Elsevier, Inc. All rights reserved.

Drugs Used to Treat Diabetes Mellitus

Answer Key: Textbook page references are provided as a guide for answering these questions. A complete answer key is provided to your instructor.

MATCHING

Match the key terms on the left with the definitions on the right.

Key Terms

1. _____ hypoglycemia
2. _____ paresthesia
3. _____ prediabetes
4. _____ gestational diabetes mellitus (GDM)
5. _____ type 1 diabetes mellitus
6. _____ hyperglycemia
7. _____ microvascular complications
8. _____ type 2 diabetes mellitus
9. _____ macrovascular complications

Definitions

a. characterized by polydipsia, polyphagia, and polyuria
b. characterized by a decrease in beta cell activity, insulin resistance, or an increase in glucose production by the liver
c. a destruction of the capillaries in the eyes, kidneys, and peripheral nerves
d. blood glucose less than 70 mg/dL
e. atherosclerosis of the middle to large arteries causing strokes, MIs, and peripheral vascular disease
f. characterized by abnormal glucose tolerance during pregnancy
g. a condition in which patients who are normally euglycemic, develop hyperglycemia when challenged with an oral glucose tolerance test
h. numbness and tingling of the extremities
i. fasting plasma glucose level of greater than 100 mg/dL

REVIEW QUESTIONS

Scenario #1: A 73-year-old patient came to the outpatient clinic complaining of left great toe being painful, swollen, and red. The patient has a history of type 2 diabetes mellitus, asthma, atrial fibrillation, peripheral arterial disease, gastric bypass surgery, and neuropathy.

Objective: Identify the major nursing considerations associated with the management of the patient with diabetes (e.g., nutritional evaluation, laboratory values, activity and exercise, and psychological considerations).

NCLEX item type: multiple response
Cognitive skill: generate solutions

10. The nurse reviewed the medical nutrition therapy recommended for patients with diabetes, and knows it includes which recommendations? *(Select all that apply.)* **(565)**
    1. Eliminating all sugar from the diet
    2. Weight loss is recommended for all adults with BMI > 25
    3. Use of the new system called the *consistent carbohydrate diabetes meal plan*
    4. Use of only the approved artificial sweeteners as sugar substitutes
    5. Limiting alcoholic drinks to two daily for men and one daily for women

Copyright © 2023 by Elsevier, Inc. All rights reserved.

NCLEX item type: cloze
Cognitive skill: recognize cues
Choose the most likely options for the information missing from the statements below by selecting from the list of options provided.

11. The nurse instructed the patient in scenario #1 on glucose testing and explained that _____1_____is an important lab to monitor because it will reflect _____2___, while ____1_____is the value tested during times of stress, when there is an infection or when _____2_____is suspected. *(573-574)*

Option 1	Option 2
Fructosamine	The glucose control over the past 2 to 3 months
Ketones in the urine	Hyperglycemia
Blood glucose	Hypoglycemia
Glycosylated hemoglobin or A1C	The presence of renal disease

NCLEX item type: multiple response
Cognitive skill: application

12. The nurse was concerned about the psychological considerations of the patients in the scenario #1 with type 2 diabetes. Which statements by the nurse are therapeutic and can help the patient adjust? *(Select all that apply.)* *(570)*
    1. "The diagnosis of diabetes is a lot to take in, what concerns you the most?"
    2. "Learning about the management of diabetes takes time and it is best to approach it as a long-term commitment."
    3. "This should not be a problem, it involves taking insulin every day and testing blood glucose levels."
    4. "Let's talk about what activities you routinely do and your work schedule."
    5. "If you change your diet and lose weight I am sure your diabetes will be controlled."

NCLEX item type: multiple response
Cognitive skill: evaluate

13. The nurse is educating the patient in scenario #1 about activity and exercise, and because of neuropathy, recommended which types of exercises? *(Select all that apply.)* *(571)*
    1. Walking
    2. Bicycling
    3. Swimming
    4. Rowing
    5. Treadmill

Objective: Compare the signs and symptoms of hypoglycemia and hyperglycemia.
NCLEX item type: multiple choice
Cognitive skill: interpret

14. A nurse was discussing the symptoms and management of hypoglycemia with the patient in scenario #1. Which statement by the patient would indicate that further education is needed? *(573)*
    1. "When I start to feel hungry, get a headache, and my vision blurs, I know I am getting hypoglycemic."
    2. "When I start to feel hypoglycemic, I should drink some fruit juice with sugar added."
    3. "I can control the episodes of hypoglycemia by eating at regular times and watching what I eat."
    4. "I know I am getting hypoglycemic when I start to feel sleepy shortly after eating a large meal."

NCLEX item type: multiple choice
Cognitive skill: constrast

15. A nurse caring for a diabetic patient noted the following symptoms: headache, nausea and vomiting, rapid pulse, and shallow respirations. What condition could this represent? *(573)*
    1. Insulin overdose
    2. Hypoglycemia
    3. Hyperglycemia
    4. Paresthesias

NCLEX item type: multiple response
Cognitive skill: explain

16. The nurse educated the patient on the causes of hyperglycemia. Which conditions will the nurse discuss? *(Select all that apply.)* *(573)*
    1. Overeating
    2. Vomiting
    3. Acute illness
    4. Infections
    5. Diarrhea

Objective: Describe the action and use of insulin to control diabetes mellitus.
NCLEX item type: multiple choice
Cognitive skill: knowledge

17. The nurse educates the patient in scenario #1 on the type of insulin that has an onset of 1–2 hours, peaks within 4-12 hours, and lasts from 14 to 24 hours. Which type of insulin is the nurse discussing? *(576)*
    1. Intermediate-acting
    2. Short-acting
    3. Rapid-acting
    4. Long-acting

NCLEX item type: multiple choice
Cognitive skill: comprehension

18. The nurse was teaching the patient the ideal time to administer rapid-acting insulin. Which time interval is correct? *(576)*
    1. 30 minutes before a meal
    2. 30 minutes after a meal
    3. Within 10–15 minutes of a meal
    4. Immediately after a meal

Copyright © 2023 by Elsevier, Inc. All rights reserved.

NCLEX item type: grid/matrix
Cognitive skill: analyze cues
19. The nurse compared the different insulins and their actions and considerations. Indicate with an 'X' which insulin has the following actions and considerations. *(576)*

Actions and considerations	Rapid acting	Short acting	Intermediate acting	Long acting
Peaks within 30 minutes				
Given with meals				
Decrease the blood sugar level rapidly				
No large fluctuations in insulin levels will occur				
Usually administered 30–60 minutes before meals				
Commonly administered in the evening				
Can be given intravenously				
Cannot be mixed with other insulins				

NCLEX item type: multiple choice
Cognitive skill: evaluate
20. The nurse is educating the patient in the scenario on the use of the rapid-acting insulin aspart while in the hospital and knows more education is needed after the patient makes which remark? *(576)*
   1. "This insulin has an onset of 1-2 hours and lasts 16 hours."
   2. "I need to have my blood sugar checked four times a day with this insulin."
   3. "The insulin aspart that I am receiving is a rapid-acting one that peaks in 1–2 hours."
   4. "So as I understand it, I will only be on insulin while I am in the hospital to control my blood sugar."

Scenario #2: A patient recently diagnoses with type 2 diabetes attended a nurse lead patient education session on diabetic management that discussed, lifestyle changes, activity, diet, and medications.

Objective: Discuss the action and use of oral hypoglycemic agents to control diabetes mellitus.
NCLEX item type: multiple choice
Cognitive skill: classify
21. The nurse explains to the patient in scenario #2 that the oral hypoglycemic agent they are taking will lower blood sugar in diabetic patients by increasing the sensitivity of muscle and fat tissue to insulin. Which class of oral hypoglycemic agents does this describe? *(584)*
   1. Meglitinides
   2. Thiazolidinediones
   3. Sulfonylureas
   4. Incretin mimetic agents

NCLEX item type: multiple choice
Cognitive skill: explain
22. The nurse discussed with the patient in scenario #2 that it is important to know the adverse effects that may occur with oral hypoglycemic agents. Which statement by the patient indicates further education is needed? *(583-584)*
   1. "The drug repaglinide that I am taking should not cause any hypoglycemia unless I have to take certain medications that will interact with it."
   2. "I am taking repaglinide with metformin to help me control my glucose."
   3. "The medication I am taking, repaglinide works by stimulating the pancreas to produce more insulin."
   4. "It is important to check my blood sugar when I am taking any NSAIDs with this medication since it may lower my sugar levels."

NCLEX item type: multiple choice
Cognitive skill: compare
23. The nurse recognizes that alpha-glucosidase inhibitors are an example of the type of oral hypoglycemic agent that works by lowering blood sugar in diabetic patients by what mechanism of action? *(586)*
   1. These agents increase the sensitivity of muscle and fat tissue to insulin.
   2. These agents inhibit digestive enzymes that result in delayed glucose absorption.
   3. These agents stimulate the release of insulin from the beta cells of the pancreas.
   4. These agents enhance insulin secretion and suppressing glucagon secretion from the liver.

Copyright © 2023 by Elsevier, Inc. All rights reserved.

NCLEX item type: multiple choice
Cognitive skill: knowledge

24. The nurse realized the patient in scenario #1 was having difficulty managing their diabetes because the A1C level result was what? *(566)*
    1. 5.3%
    2. 6.0%
    3. 8.5%
    4. 4.0%

NCLEX item type: multiple choice
Cognitive skill: interpret

25. The patient in scenario #1 was being started on glipizide (Glucotrol). Which statement by the nurse would be included in the discussion of adverse effects from these drugs? *(582)*
    1. "If you develop a rash with itching, don't worry; it should get better eventually."
    2. "You will need to change your diet with these drugs and consume greater portions of protein."
    3. "You may experience nausea, vomiting, and abdominal cramps, in which case you must stop taking the drug immediately."
    4. "You may develop abdominal cramps and diarrhea, but these symptoms will resolve with continued use of your medication."

NCLEX item type: multiple choice
Cognitive skill: classify

26. It is important for the nurse to inform female patients with diabetes that an alternative method of birth control should be used when taking which oral hypoglycemic agent? *(585)*
    1. miglitol
    2. glyburide
    3. empaglifozsin (Jardiance)
    4. pioglitazone (Actos)

Objective: Discuss the educational needs for patients with complications from diabetes.

NCLEX item type: multiple response
Cognitive skill: application

27. The nurse discussed with the patient in scenario #2 the signs and symptoms of microvascular complications of peripheral vascular disease. Which statements by the nurse are included in the discussion? *(Select all that apply.)* *(564)*
    1. "If you find you have pain in your legs with exercise that is relieved with rest, this is a complication called claudication."
    2. "You may find that urinary tract infections may increase in frequency as a complication."
    3. "The skin over the legs, hands, fingers, and feet may have a reddish-blue discoloration as a complication."
    4. "You may notice that temperature of the skin in your feet and legs may be cool to the touch."
    5. "It is important to prevent complications such as ulcers, injury and infections to the legs with meticulous regular care."

NCLEX item type: multiple response
Cognitive skill: compare

28. The patient in scenario #1 had examples of complications from diabetes. Which conditions are complications? *(Select all that apply.)* *(564)*
    1. Asthma
    2. Neuropathy
    3. Atrial fibrillation
    4. Peripheral arterial disease
    5. Cellulitis of the great toe

NCLEX item type: multiple response
Cognitive skill: analyze

29. The nurse recognizes that major macrovascular complications of diabetes are associated with atherosclerotic disease of the middle to large arteries which often lead to myocardial infarction and stroke. Complications of diabetes include both micro and macrovascular processes and include which conditions? *(Select all that apply.)* *(564)*
    1. Retinopathy leading to blindness
    2. Ototoxicity leading to hearing loss
    3. Nonhealing ulcers leading to amputations of the lower extremities
    4. Renal disease leading to end-stage renal disease and dialysis
    5. Neuropathies leading to bladder incontinence and gastroparesis

NCLEX item type: multiple response
Cognitive skill: generate solutions

30. Which statements does the nurse include when teaching health promotion activities to a patient with type 1 diabetes mellitus? *(Select all that apply.)* *(570-573)*
    1. "If you feel sick, cut your insulin dose by half."
    2. "Meal planning is important and getting consistent carbohydrates is recommended."
    3. "Self-monitoring of your blood glucose is advised when exercising."
    4. "Notify your primary healthcare provider immediately if you are unable to keep anything down."
    5. "Extra insulin is often needed to meet the demands of illness, so be aware of the development of hyperglycemia, which is common in patients with acute illness, injury, or surgery."

Copyright © 2023 by Elsevier, Inc. All rights reserved.

Student Name_____   Date_____

Drugs Used to Treat Thyroid Disease

Answer Key: Textbook page references are provided as a guide for answering these questions. A complete answer key is provided to your instructor.

MATCHING

Match the definition on the right with the key term on the left. Definitions may be used more than once.

Key Term

1. _____ myxedema
2. _____ cretinism
3. _____ hyperthyroidism
4. _____ thyrotoxicosis
5. _____ hypothyroidism
6. _____ triiodothyronine
7. _____ thyroxine

Definition

a. congenital hypothyroidism
b. excess production of thyroid hormones
c. thyroid hormone
d. inadequate thyroid hormone production
e. thickened, non-pitting edematous changes to the soft tissues
f. excessive formation of thyroid hormones and their secretion into the circulatory system

REVIEW QUESTIONS

Scenario #1: A 48-year-old female patient came to an outpatient clinic complaining of increased fatigue and unexplained weight gain. She mentioned that she was beginning to have problems with constipation and felt cold all the time.

Objective: Describe the signs, symptoms, drugs, and nursing interventions associated with hypothyroidism.

NCLEX item type: multiple choice
Cognitive skill: knowledge

8. A patient with dramatic weight loss and rapid, bounding pulse may be suffering from what disorder? *(598)*
   1. Cretinism
   2. Myxedema
   3. Hypothyroidism
   4. Hyperthyroidism

NCLEX item type: multiple response
Cognitive skill: application

9. What focused assessments should be performed by the nurse for the patient in scenario #1 suspected of having hypothyroidism? *(Select all that apply.)* *(599)*
   1. Determine if there has been any weight changes over past 3 months
   2. Observe for eyelid retraction or exophthalmos
   3. Assess degree of alertness and pace of responsiveness
   4. Ask about any ringing in the ear or loss of hearing
   5. Note bradycardia or tachycardia and any palpitations

NCLEX item type: multiple choice
Cognitive skill: interpret

10. The nurse educates the patient in scenario #1 with hypothyroidism regarding dietary changes. Which statement by the nurse needs to be corrected? *(600)*
    1. "Your healthcare provider will likely order a low-calorie diet for you at this time."
    2. "It is important to make sure you take plenty of fluids daily unless comorbidities prohibit it."
    3. "Your diet should include high-calorie since you are having a fast metabolism."
    4. "It is important to have an adequate amount of fiber in your diet with bran and fresh fruits."

Copyright © 2023 by Elsevier, Inc. All rights reserved.

NCLEX item type: multiple choice
Cognitive skill: classify
11. The nurse expects the patient in scenario #1 needs to be started on a thyroid replacement hormone such as which drug? *(601)*
    1. methimazole
    2. propylthiouracil
    3. levothyroxine
    4. thyroglobulin

NCLEX item type: multiple response
Cognitive skill: application
12. The patient in scenario #1 was diagnosed with hypothyroidism and the nurse gave which instructions regarding this diagnosis and treatment? *(Select all that apply.)* *(601)*
    1. "You should take your Synthroid with food around lunchtime."
    2. "You will need to start taking thyroid hormones for the treatment of this condition."
    3. "You may find that you will be more comfortable in a warm environment."
    4. "You need to be aware of the signs of hyperthyroidism, which can be caused by too much thyroid medication."
    5. "The dosages of this thyroid medication start high and then gradually decrease in amount until you reach your daily maintenance dose."

Scenario #2: A patient came to the clinic with complaints of weight loss, despite increased appetite and feeling hot all the time, with increase in sweating. The patient also noted having tremors starting in the hands.

Objective: Describe the signs, symptoms, drugs, and nursing interventions associated with hyperthyroidism.
NCLEX item type: grid/matrix
Cognitive skill: recognize cues
13. The nurse reviewed the conditions that cause thyroid disorders. Indicate with an 'X' the conditions that cause hypothyroidism, and those that cause hyperthyroidism. *(597-598)*

	Hypothyroidism	Hyperthyroidism
Thyroid surgery		
Nodular goiter		
Thyroiditis		
Radiation exposure		
Tumors of the pituitary gland		
Graves' disease		
Thyroid carcinoma		
Acute viral thyroiditis		

NCLEX item type: multiple response
Cognitive skill: application
14. Which manifestation does the nurse expect to find upon assessing the patient in scenario #2 who has been diagnosed with hyperthyroidism? *(Select all that apply.)* *(598)*
    1. Lethargy
    2. Constipation
    3. Weight loss
    4. Rapid, bounding pulse
    5. Nervousness and agitation

NCLEX item type: multiple response
Cognitive skill: classify
15. The primary therapeutic outcome for drug therapy for patients with hyperthyroidism is a gradual return to normal thyroid metabolic function expected from which drugs? *(Select all that apply.)* *(602-603)*
    1. iodine-131
    2. levothyroxine
    3. liothyronine
    4. propylthiouracil
    5. methimazole

NCLEX item type: multiple choice
Cognitive skill: interpret
16. The nurse has been teaching a patient in scenario #2 diagnosed with hyperthyroidism about proper nutritional habits to follow. Which patient statement indicates a need for further teaching? *(599-600)*
    1. "I know I need to reduce fiber in my diet."
    2. "I will drink decaffeinated cola."
    3. "If I get diarrhea, I will eat bran products, fruits and fresh vegetables."
    4. "I will eat a high-calorie diet, about 4000–5000 calories a day."

NCLEX item type: multiple choice
Cognitive skill: interpret
17. The nurse is instructing the patient in scenario #2 recently diagnosed with hyperthyroidism on an environment that best suits their needs. Which statement by the patient would indicate that further teaching is needed? *(600)*
    1. "I will try to keep my home a bit cooler even though I am not sure if my spouse will okay with that."
    2. "It should not matter what the environment is, I am sure I can take it."
    3. "So apparently I need to have a quiet, structured environment since my body cannot respond to change."
    4. "I will try to avoid stressful, anxiety-producing situation as they may make me feel worse."

Copyright © 2023 by Elsevier, Inc. All rights reserved.

Objective: Discuss the drug interactions associated with thyroid hormones and antithyroid medicines.

NCLEX item type: multiple choice
Cognitive skill: explain

18. The patient in scenario #1 was on digoxin (Lanoxin) and needed to be started on levothyroxine (Synthroid) for the treatment of hypothyroidism. Which statement by the nurse explains the interaction between these two drugs? *(602)*
    1. "You will most likely require a decreased dose of digoxin."
    2. "You will most likely require an increased dose of digoxin."
    3. "You will most likely require increasing dosages of Synthroid."
    4. "You will most likely have to adjust your dosages of Synthroid every week."

NCLEX item type: multiple choice
Cognitive skill: comprehension

19. The nurse knows that iodine-131 (^{131}I) is used in the treatment of hyperthyroidism because this drug will have what effect? *(602)*
    1. It will cause the thyroid gland to radiate a soft, warm glow.
    2. It will increase the circulating thyrotropin-releasing hormone.
    3. It will absorb all of the excess thyroid hormone that is circulating in the blood.
    4. It will be absorbed into the thyroid gland and destroy the hyperactive tissue.

NCLEX item type: multiple response
Cognitive skill: application

20. When administering iodine-131 (^{131}I) to a patient, what actions does the nurse take? *(Select all that apply.) (603)*
    1. Avoids spilling the medication
    2. Changes the patient's bedding after each dose
    3. Wears latex gloves when administering the drug
    4. Adds the medication to water and has the patient swallow it
    5. Maintains hazardous medication precautions when working with the drug

NCLEX item type: multiple choice
Cognitive skill: illustrate

21. The nurse knows that antithyroid drugs work by interfering with what? *(603)*
    1. The metabolic requirements of the body
    2. The release of thyroid hormones from the thyroid gland
    3. The formation of the hormones produced by the thyroid gland
    4. Release of thyroid-stimulating hormone from the pituitary gland.

Copyright © 2023 by Elsevier, Inc. All rights reserved.

Corticosteroids

Answer Key: Textbook page references are provided as a guide for answering these questions. A complete answer key is provided to your instructor.

MATCHING

Match the brand name drug on the right with the generic drug name on the left.

Generic Drug Name

1. _____ fluocinonide
2. _____ budesonide
3. _____ dexamethasone
4. _____ hydrocortisone
5. _____ methylprednisolone
6. _____ prednisolone
7. _____ triamcinolone

Brand Name Drug

a. Kenalog
b. Vanos
c. Cortef
d. Pediapred
e. Solu-Medrol
f. Decadron
g. Entocort

REVIEW QUESTIONS

Scenario #1: A 75-year-old patient was admitted to the hospital for respiratory failure and was diagnosed with pneumonia. The patient's history includes chronic obstructive pulmonary disease (COPD), osteoporosis, hypothyroidism, depression, congestive heart failure (CHF), coronary artery disease with previous bypass grafts, and rheumatoid arthritis. The patient's medication list includes levothyroxine, metoprolol, prednisone, duloxetine, acetaminophen, senna, and oxycodone.

Objective: Discuss the normal actions of mineralocorticoids and glucocorticoids in the body.
NCLEX item type: cloze
Cognitive skill: recognize cues
Choose the most likely options for the information missing from the statements below by selecting from the list of options provided.

8. The nurse knows that the adrenal gland secretes hormones that maintain _____1_____and regulate metabolism of_____1_____.
   These hormones are known collectively as _____2_____. *(607)*

Option 1	Option 2
Fluid and electrolyte balance	Corticosteroids
Excretion of medications	Aldosterone
Carbohydrates, fats, and protein	Mineralocorticoids
Temperature regulation	Glucocorticoids

NCLEX item type: multiple response
Cognitive skill: application

9. The corticosteroids are used to regulate the body's metabolism. Which laboratory tests will the nurse be monitoring for patients receiving these medications? *(Select all that apply.)* *(608)*
   1. Glucose
   2. Protime
   3. Calcium
   4. Potassium
   5. Sodium

NCLEX item type: multiple choice
Cognitive skill: relate

10. The nurse is teaching the patient in scenario #1 with rheumatoid arthritis about the use of glucocorticoids. Which statement by the patient indicates a need for further instruction? *(611)*
    1. "This drug has cured my disease."
    2. "This drug is relieving the inflammation associated with rheumatoid arthritis."
    3. "Although it would be great if my fingers would change back to their normal shape with this drug, I know that will not happen."
    4. "I must be aware that I am more susceptible to infections when taking these drugs."

Scenario #2: A patient with Addison disease come to the clinic for prescription renewal. The patient has been taking fludrocortisone and needs to have blood tests for follow up.

Copyright © 2023 by Elsevier, Inc. All rights reserved.

Objective: Identify the baseline assessments needed for a patient receiving corticosteroids.

NCLEX item type: multiple response
Cognitive skill: application

11. The nurse will perform a baseline assessment on the patient in scenario #1 who was prescribed methyl-prednisolone while in the hospital? *(Select all that apply.)* **(612)**
    1. Check electrolyte values
    2. Assess for dehydration
    3. Record temperature
    4. Pulse checks in supine and sitting position
    5. Orientation to date, time, and place

NCLEX item type: multiple response
Cognitive skill: evaluate outcomes

12. What are the therapeutic outcomes the nurse will expect when caring for the patient in scenario #2 on fludrocortisone therapy for Addison disease? **(611)**
    1. Controlling pulse rate
    2. Preventing weight gain
    3. Restoring fluid and electrolytes
    4. Controlling blood pressure
    5. Reducing inflammation

NCLEX item type: multiple response
Cognitive skill: application

13. The nurse is assessing the patient in scenario #1 taking glucocorticoids for the treatment of rheumatoid arthritis. Which findings are indications that the medication is exerting its desired effect? *(Select all that apply.)* **(611)**
    1. Pain relief
    2. Increased energy
    3. Relief of swelling
    4. Elevated sedimentation rates
    5. Normalization of preexisting joint deformities

NCLEX item type: multiple response
Cognitive skill: evaluate cues

14. Which signs of dehydration need to be assessed by the nurse when patients are receiving corticosteroids? *(Select all that apply.)* **(608)**
    1. Poor skin turgor
    2. Bounding pulses
    3. Peripheral edema
    4. Delayed capillary refill
    5. Sticky oral mucous membranes

Objective: Discuss the clinical uses and potential adverse effects associated with corticosteroids.

NCLEX item type: multiple choice
Cognitive skill: interpret

15. A nurse was teaching the patient in scenario #2 with Addison disease about the condition and how it is treated. Which statement by the patient indicates that further teaching is needed? **(611)**
    1. "I understand that I need to watch my weight and report significant changes."
    2. "I understand that my adrenal glands are not producing enough of the hormone needed to regulate water and electrolytes."
    3. "I know that when I go get my blood drawn, the most important test reported is the level of calcium."
    4. "I know I cannot stop taking these hormones unless I am under a healthcare provider's care."

NCLEX item type: extended multiple response
Cognitive skill: recognize cues

16. The nurse reviews the types of illnesses or conditions that are frequently treated with glucocorticoids. Which conditions are glucocorticoids effective for treating? *(Select all that apply.)* **(611)**
    1. Severe hay fever
    2. Bacterial infections
    3. Organ transplant
    4. Appendicitis
    5. Dermatomyositis
    6. Lupus erythematosus
    7. Acute constipation
    8. Rheumatoid arthritis
    9. Status asthmaticus
    10. Heart failure

NCLEX item type: multiple response
Cognitive skill: analyze cues

17. The nurse reviews the adverse effects of glucocorticoids that the patient in scenario #1 was receiving. Which effects are important to monitor for with patients who are receiving glucocorticoids such as prednisone? *(Select all that apply.)* **(613)**
    1. Hyperglycemia
    2. Hypoglycemia
    3. Peptic ulcer formation
    4. Signs of infection
    5. Electrolyte imbalances and edema

Copyright © 2023 by Elsevier, Inc. All rights reserved.

NCLEX item type: multiple choice
Cognitive skill: analyze

18. The nurse was teaching a patient about precautions necessary when receiving steroid therapy. Further education is needed when the patient makes which statement? *(610)*
    1. "I know I should not suddenly stop taking these medications."
    2. "I will need to get an identification bracelet to wear at all times."
    3. "I can expect that a weight gain of 2 pounds in 2 days is normal."
    4. "I understand that if I start to develop edema in my feet, ankles, or legs, I need to notify my healthcare provider."

NCLEX item type: multiple choice
Cognitive skill: knowledge

19. The drug prednisone (a glucocorticoid) has an antiinflammatory effect and is used for the patient in scenario #1 for which diagnosis? *(611)*
    1. Hypothyroidism
    2. Rheumatoid arthritis
    3. Depression
    4. Osteoporosis

NCLEX item type: multiple response
Cognitive skill: application

20. The nurse recognized that glucocorticoids must be used with caution in patients with which disorders? *(Select all that apply.)* *(613)*
    1. Diabetes mellitus
    2. Peptic ulcer disease
    3. Upper respiratory infections
    4. Heart failure
    5. Mental disturbances

Copyright © 2023 by Elsevier, Inc. All rights reserved.

Gonadal Hormones

Answer Key: Textbook page references are provided as a guide for answering these questions. A complete answer key is provided to your instructor.

MATCHING
Match the brand name drug on the right with the generic drug name on the left.

Generic Drug Name

1. _____ esterified estrogen
2. _____ testosterone gel
3. _____ conjugated estrogen
4. _____ norethindrone
5. _____ estradiol
6. _____ methyltestosterone

Brand Name Drug

a. Aygestin
b. Estrace
c. Premarin
d. AndroGel
e. Methitest
f. Menest

REVIEW QUESTIONS
Scenario #1: A 35 year-old female recently tried to stop taking their medications because she did not believe they were working, started to have symptoms again and came in to the clinic.

Objective: Identify the uses of estrogens and progestins.
NCLEX item type: multiple response
Cognitive skill: application
7. The nurse interviewing the patient in scenario #1 who came to the clinic to get their prescription renewed, noted that they were using progestin therapy. What conditions are generally treated with progestin? *(Select all that apply.)* **(620)**
    1. Severe acne
    2. Endometriosis
    3. Secondary amenorrhea
    4. Breakthrough uterine bleeding
    5. Hot flash symptoms of menopause

NCLEX item type: multiple response
Cognitive skill: application
8. The nurse recognizes the therapeutic uses for estrogen therapy. Which conditions are estrogens used for ? *(Select all that apply.)* **(617)**
    1. Treating severe acne in males
    2. Preventing osteoporosis
    3. Providing contraception
    4. Slowing the disease process of advanced prostate cancer
    5. Relieving hot flash symptoms of menopause

Copyright © 2023 by Elsevier, Inc. All rights reserved.

NCLEX item type: cloze
Cognitive skill: recognize cues
Choose the most likely options for the information missing from the statements below by selecting from the list of options provided.

9. The nurse explains the uses of estrogens such as _____1_____ to the patient in scenario #1 and mentioned that they are contraindicated in patients who _____2_____because of the potential for ____3_____. *(618)*

Option 1	Option 2	Option 3
Provera	Are recovering postpartum	Birth defects
Premarin	Have advanced prostate cancer	Excess uterine bleeding
Aygestin	Are in the early stages of pregnancy	Developing seizures
Methitest	Are in the process of menopause	Thromboembolic disorders

Scenario #2: A 29-year-old male with hypogonadism comes into the clinic complaining of muscle cramps, tremors, and feeling tired. It was determined that he was experiencing an electrolyte imbalance from his medication.

Objective: Compare the adverse effects seen with the use of estrogen hormones with those seen with androgens.
NCLEX item type: multiple choice
Cognitive skill: analyze

10. While assessing a female patient on estrogen therapy for birth control, which adverse effect does the nurse report to the healthcare provider? *(618)*
    1. Nausea
    2. Weight gain
    3. Breast tenderness
    4. Breakthrough bleeding

NCLEX item type: multiple choice
Cognitive skill: constrast

11. The nurse expects that hormone therapy will be used for palliative treatment in patients with prostate cancer. Which gonadal hormone therapy will be used in this case? *(618)*
    1. Thyroid therapy
    2. Progestin therapy
    3. Androgen therapy
    4. Estrogen therapy

NCLEX item type: multiple response
Cognitive skill: application

12. The nurse is teaching the patient in scenario #2 to report which effects of methyltestosterone to report to their healthcare provider? *(Select all that apply.)* *(622)*
    1. Masculinization
    2. Gastric irritation
    3. Jaundice, anorexia
    4. Weight gain of more than 2 pounds in a week
    5. Pain, edema, warmth, and erythema in the lower leg

NCLEX item type: multiple response
Cognitive skill: evaluate cues

13. Drug interactions are important to monitor for patients on more than one classification of medications. The nurse will determine if there is a concern with patients started on estrogens who are also on what other medication? *(Select all that apply.)* *(618)*
    1. Rifampin and estrogens may cause jaundice.
    2. Insulin and estrogens may cause hypoglycemia.
    3. Warfarin and estrogens may result in risk for clotting.
    4. Thyroid hormones and estrogens may cause hypothyroidism.
    5. Phenytoin and estrogens may reduce contraceptive activity.

NCLEX item type: multiple response
Cognitive skill: application

14. The nurse discusses with the patient in scenario #1 the serious adverse effects that may be experienced with progestins. Which conditions are serious adverse effects that need to be reported? *(Select all that apply.)* *(621)*
    1. Severe acne
    2. Depression
    3. Cholestatic jaundice
    4. Continuous headache
    5. Weight gain and edema

NCLEX item type: multiple response
Cognitive skill: interpret

15. The patient in scenario #2 is ordered testosterone gel every 24 hours. The nurse teaches the patient to rotate the application sites for the patch to which areas of the body? *(Select all that apply.)* *(621)*
    1. Hips
    2. Abdomen
    3. Shoulders
    4. Upper arms
    5. Scrotum

Copyright © 2023 by Elsevier, Inc. All rights reserved.

NCLEX item type: multiple response
Cognitive skill: generate solutions
16. The nurse is teaching the patient in scenario #2 about ways to minimize the adverse effects of androgen therapy, which include what suggestions? *(Select all that apply.)* **(623)**
    1. "You should drink 8–12 glasses of water a day."
    2. "You should chew and swallow the buccal tablet."
    3. "You should include weight-bearing exercises in your ADLs."
    4. "You should report any weight gain of more than 2 pounds per week."
    5. "You should notify the prescriber if nausea, anorexia, and jaundice occur."

NCLEX item type: multiple response
Cognitive skill: application
17. The nurse is teaching a patient about the adverse effects of estrogen therapy. Which statement by the patient indicates a need for further teaching? **(618)**
    1. "Weight gain is a common adverse effect of estrogen therapy."
    2. "Breast tenderness is to be expected when I start this drug."
    3. "Low blood pressure is a common side effect of estrogen therapy."
    4. "If I experience any breakthrough bleeding between my menstrual periods, I will notify my primary care provider immediately."

NCLEX item type: multiple response
Cognitive skill: recognize cues
18. The nurse recognizes that when androgens are given to female patients that the adverse effect of masculinization may occur. Which symptoms are seen with masculinization? *(Select all that apply.)* **(623)**
    1. Deepening voice
    2. Gastric irritation
    3. Clearing of acne
    4. Menstrual irregularity
    5. Growth of facial hair

NCLEX item type: grid/matrix
Cognitive skill: recognize cues
19. The nurse reviews the uses for androgens and compares them to the effects of estrogens when discussing gonadal hormones with a student nurse. Indicate with an 'X' the conditions that androgens are used to treat and the effects that estrogens have. **617,621**

	Androgens used to treat	Estrogens have these effects
Release of gonadotropins		
Wasting syndrome associated with AIDS		
Palliation of breast cancer		
Fluid retention		
Hypogonadism		
Regulate protein metabolism.		
Androgen deficiency		
Elevated blood sugars		

Copyright © 2023 by Elsevier, Inc. All rights reserved.

Drugs Used in Obstetrics

Answer Key: Textbook page references are provided as a guide for answering these questions. A complete answer key is provided to your instructor.

MATCHING

Match the drug name on the right with the correct usage for the drug on the left.

Usage for Drug

1. _____ used to inhibit premature labor

2. _____ used to induce labor at term

3. _____ used to expel uterine contents

4. _____ used as an antidote for magnesium intoxication

5. _____ prevents vitamin K deficiency bleeding of the newborn

6. _____ used to stimulate uterine contractions

Drug

a. phytonadione
b. dinoprostone
c. methylergonovine maleate
d. oxytocin
e. magnesium sulfate
f. calcium gluconate

REVIEW QUESTIONS

Scenario #1: A 32-year-old gravida 1, para 0 was admitted after 38 weeks gestation to the local delivery unit in possible labor. After the initial assessment, the patient was noted to have high blood pressure, pedal edema, and hyper-reflexia. The patient was diagnosed with preeclampsia and was started on a magnesium sulfate infusion.

Objective: Identify appropriate nursing assessments during normal labor and delivery.
NCLEX item type: multiple response
Cognitive skill: application

7. The nurse needs to be aware of which potential obstetric complications in pregnant women? *(Select all that apply.) (626)*
   1. Infection
   2. Preterm labor
   3. Hypoglycemia
   4. Gestational diabetes
   5. Premature rupture of membranes

NCLEX item type: multiple choice
Cognitive skill: knowledge

8. The nurse was discussing postpartum care with a new mother and knew that more teaching was needed after the mother made which statement? *(634-635)*
   1. "I understand that my baby will gain about 1 ounce per day until day 5."
   2. "I can take a mild analgesic 40 minutes before breastfeeding."
   3. "I know I need to continue to eat a well-balanced diet when breastfeeding."
   4. "If I note any foul odor from my vaginal discharge, I know to call my healthcare provider."

NCLEX item type: multiple response
Cognitive skill: illustrate

9. What are routine nursing assessments performed on pregnant women no matter what trimester they are in? *(Select all that apply.) (626)*
   1. Weight
   2. Blood pressure
   3. Vaginal exams
   4. Hemoglobin and hematocrit
   5. Fundal height and fetal heart sounds

Copyright © 2023 by Elsevier, Inc. All rights reserved.

NCLEX item type: multiple response
Cognitive skill: evaluate
10. The nurse will perform an assessment of pregnant woman which includes obtaining an obstetric history. What questions will the nurse ask? *(Select all that apply.)* *(625)*
   1. "How many children do you have? And how many times have you been pregnant?"
   2. "Have any of your previous deliveries been by cesarean?"
   3. "What medications are you currently taking?"
   4. "Have any of your children been premature at birth?"
   5. "Have you ever had a stillbirth? Or a spontaneous or therapeutic abortion?"

Objective: Discuss potential complications of preterm labor and when uterine relaxants and magnesium sulfate are used.
NCLEX item type: multiple response
Cognitive skill: application
11. The nurse reviewed the primary clinical indications for the use of uterine stimulants. Which situations warrant the use of uterine stimulants such as oxytocin? *(Select all that apply.)* *(636)*
   1. Suppression of lactation
   2. Induction of therapeutic abortion
   3. Induction or augmentation of labor
   4. Control of postsurgical hemorrhage
   5. During preeclampsia to induce labor
NCLEX item type: multiple choice
Cognitive skill: compare
12. The nurse discusses with the patient in scenario #1 the reasons for the use of uterine relaxants on the pregnant uterus? *(636-637)*
   1. Uterine relaxants are used to induce or augment labor.
   2. Uterine relaxants are used to control postpartum hemorrhage.
   3. Uterine relaxants are used to suppress the flow of colostrum.
   4. Uterine relaxants are used to delay or prevent labor and delivery in selected patients.
NCLEX item type: multiple choice
Cognitive skill: interpret
13. Which assessment findings that the nurse obtained from the patient in scenario #1 would indicate that the magnesium sulfate infusion should be discontinued? *(640-641)*
   1. Absence of deep tendon reflexes
   2. Respiratory rate of 16 breaths/min
   3. Urinary output of 45 mL during the past hour
   4. Decrease in blood pressure from 180/100 to 150/90 mm Hg

NCLEX item type: multiple choice
Cognitive skill: knowledge
14. The nurse knows to perform which interventionwhen a pregnant woman is in preterm labor? *(630-631)*
   1. Restrict fluids
   2. Position the patient on her back
   3. Administer uterine stimulants
   4. Administer uterine relaxants
NCLEX item type: multiple choice
Cognitive skill: comprehension
15. The nurse recognized the signs of fetal distress when monitoring a mother in labor. Which change in heart rate indicates the fetus is in distress? *(638)*
   1. Fetal heart rate 120–160 beats/min following any contraction
   2. Fetal heart rate >160 beats/min lasting less than 10 seconds after contractions
   3. Fetal heart rate 140 beats/min lasting longer than 15 seconds after contractions
   4. Fetal heart rate >160 followed by heart rate <120 occurring frequently following contractions

Objective: Describe assessments needed for uterine stimulants administered for induction of labor, augmentation of labor, and postpartum atony and hemorrhage.
NCLEX item type: multiple response
Cognitive skill: application
16. The nurse assesses the patient in scenario #1 receiving an infusion of oxytocin (Pitocin) to induce labor and determines the infant is in distress. Which actions does the nurse take? *(Select all that apply.)* *(638)*
   1. Turns the patient to the right lateral position
   2. Notifies the healthcare provider immediately
   3. Administers a bolus of magnesium sulfate
   4. Administers oxygen by nasal cannula or facemask
   5. Reduces the oxytocin infusion to the slowest possible rate according to hospital policy
NCLEX item type: multiple choice
Cognitive skill: analyze
17. The nurse was performing a postpartum assessment on a mother who was receiving oxytocin (Pitocin) therapy for control of bleeding and found the uterus to be boggy. What is the nurse's next action? *(638)*
   1. Massage the uterus.
   2. Administer magnesium sulfate.
   3. Slow the rate of the infusion.
   4. Call the healthcare provider immediately.

Copyright © 2023 by Elsevier, Inc. All rights reserved.

NCLEX item type: multiple choice
Cognitive skill: knowledge

18. When working with patients receiving oxytocin (Pitocin), the nurse must assess for the development of water intoxication because oxytocin therapy causes which effect? *(638)*
    1. Increased urine output
    2. Hyperalert state
    3. Extreme thirst in patients
    4. Stimulation of antidiuretic hormone

NCLEX item type: multiple response
Cognitive skill: ordering

19. List in correct order the steps to take for managing patients in preterm labor. *(628,630)*
    1. _____ Determine contraindications to tocolysis (i.e., placenta previa, fetal distress)
    2. _____ Monitor contractions and determine estimated gestational age
    3. _____ Administer indomethacin, nifedipine, or magnesium sulfate
    4. _____ Take vital signs of the mother and apply fetal monitoring
    5. _____ Observe for cervical changes

NCLEX item type: multiple choice
Cognitive skill: classify

20. A patient is receiving magnesium sulfate to inhibit preterm labor. Which drug does the nurse have readily available if magnesium toxicity should occur? *(641)*
    1. atropine
    2. epinephrine
    3. calcium gluconate
    4. potassium chloride

Scenario #2: A full term infant was delivered to a first time mother who labored for 12 hours.

Objective: Discuss education needed for care of the neonate, including erythromycin ophthalmic ointment.

NCLEX item type: multiple response
Cognitive skill: application

21. The nurse caring for the neonate in scenario #2 estimates at 1 minute and 5 minutes after delivery using the Apgar rating system, which parameters of the newborn? *(Select all that apply.)* *(629)*
    1. Heart rate
    2. Blood pressure
    3. Muscle tone
    4. Reflex irritability
    5. Color of body and extremities

NCLEX item type: multiple response
Cognitive skill: application

22. The nurse attends the delivery of a mother in labor and needs to complete which of the following procedures immediately after the birth of the newborn? *(Select all that apply.)* *(634)*
    1. Breastfeeding
    2. Eye prophylaxis
    3. Clamping the umbilical cord
    4. Determining an Apgar score
    5. Airway—suction with bulb syringe if needed

NCLEX item type: multiple choice
Cognitive skill: relate

23. The nurse explains to the mother in scenario #2 that after birth all infants have prophylactic erythromycin ointment applied to their eyes. What will this treatment prevent? *(641)*
    1. Wilms' tumor
    2. Nearsightedness
    3. Pheochromocytoma
    4. Ophthalmia neonatorum

NCLEX item type: multiple choice
Cognitive skill: explain

24. A new mother in scenario #2 asks the nurse why her newborn needs a shot of vitamin K. Which is an appropriate statement by the nurse? *(642)*
    1. "All babies get this to prevent ophthalmia neonatorum."
    2. "The delivery may have caused an infection in your baby and this will take care of it."
    3. "This will help increase the amount of natural bacteria in your baby's GI system."
    4. "Newborns are often deficient in vitamin K and we want to prevent any bleeding issues."

Copyright © 2023 by Elsevier, Inc. All rights reserved.

Drugs Used in Men's and Women's Health

Answer Key: Textbook page references are provided as a guide for answering these questions. A complete answer key is provided to your instructor.

MATCHING
Match the term on the right with the definition on the left.

Definition

1. _____ pathogens commonly transmitted by sexual contact
2. _____ an enlargement of the prostate gland
3. _____ the consistent inability to achieve or maintain an erection sufficient for satisfactory sexual activity
4. _____ an abnormal, whitish vaginal discharge that can occur at any age
5. _____ a common bone disease of low mineral density which results in bone fragility and risk of fractures
6. _____ irregular periods, infrequent periods, and spotting between periods

Term

a. leukorrhea
b. sexually transmitted infections
c. dysmenorrhea
d. osteoporosis
e. benign prostatic hyperplasia
f. erectile dysfunction

REVIEW QUESTIONS

Scenario #1: A nurse working at an outpatient clinic discussed with a women who was concerned about which type of contraceptive to take. The patient informed the nurse that she had been unsuccessful in trying to quit smoking, and recently discovered she was anemic.

Objective: Describe the major adverse effects and contraindications to the use of oral contraceptive agents.
NCLEX item type: multiple choice
Cognitive skill: evaluate

7. The nurse educated a woman on adverse effects that need to be reported from the combination pill. What instruction does the nurse need to discuss with the woman? *(654)*
   1. "The combination pill may cause nausea and needs to be reported."
   2. "You need to report if you have missed a dose."
   3. "The combination pill has been shown to cause weight gain and needs to be reported."
   4. "Any time you are having leg pain, chest pain, or feel shortness of breath while taking the combination pill you need to report it."

NCLEX item type: multiple response
Cognitive skill: application

8. The nurse discussed the possibility of the mini-pill, which only contains progestin,#1. The nurse explains that this oral contraceptive is preferred by some women because of their history of which conditions that are aggravated by estrogens? *(Select all that apply.) (652)*
   1. Diabetes
   2. Depression
   3. Migraines
   4. Hypertension
   5. Hypothyroidism

NCLEX item type: multiple choice
Cognitive skill: explain

9. The nurse explains to the woman in scenario #1 why smoking while on the pill is considered to be risky for women. Which statement would the nurse use that is accurate? *(652)*
   1. "When you take oral contraceptives and smoke it increases the chance of pregnancy."
   2. "It is not recommended to smoke and take oral contraceptives since it may increase the possibility of breakthrough bleeding."
   3. "The pill loses its effectiveness after just one cigarette."
   4. "It is not recommended to smoke and take oral contraceptives because of the increased likelihood of developing a serious blood clot."

Copyright © 2023 by Elsevier, Inc. All rights reserved.

NCLEX item type: multiple choice
Cognitive skill: knowledge

10. The nurse explained the different types of combination pills with the women in scenario #1. Which type was discussed as being used for patients who have heavy menses with associated anemia? *(652)*
    1. Biphasic
    2. Triphasic
    3. Quadriphasic
    4. Continuous cycle

NCLEX item type: multiple choice
Cognitive skill: relate

11. The nurse discussed with the women in scenario #1 the precautions that must be taken before starting on oral contraceptives. Which premedication assessment will the nurse gather? *(652-653)*
    1. Obtain a list of past sexual partners
    2. Ensure that the patient is not pregnant
    3. Determine the sperm count of the male partner
    4. Determine if any sexually transmitted infections have been contracted

NCLEX item type: grid/matrix
Cognitive skill: evaluate cues

12. The nurse knows that the minipill produces contraception differently from the combination pill. Indicate with a 'X' the actions of the minipill and the actions of the combination pill. *(650-652)*

	Minipill (progestins only)	Combination pill (estrogens and progestins)
Blocks the pituitary release of follicle-stimulating hormone		
Inhibits sperm migration		
Causes the cervical mucus to become thicker and more viscous		
Inhibits the release of luteinizing hormone		

Objective: Identify the patient teaching necessary with the administration of the transdermal contraceptive and the intravaginal hormonal contraceptive.

NCLEX item type: multiple response
Cognitive skill: recognize cues

13. In teaching a patient about the use of norelgestromin-ethinyl estradiol transdermal system (Xulane), which statements does the nurse include? *(Select all that apply.)* *(655-656)*
    1. "Do not place the patch on your breast."
    2. "Trim the patch to best fit the area where you wish to apply it."
    3. "Apply the patch to the buttock, abdomen, upper outer arm, or upper torso."
    4. "Avoid lotions or creams on the areas of the skin where the patch is applied because the patch may not adhere properly."
    5. "If the patch is partially detached for less than 24 hours, try to reapply it in the same place or replace it with a new patch immediately."

NCLEX item type: multiple choice
Cognitive skill: explain

14. A patient asks the nurse about what to do when she misses her period while on the NuvaRing. What is an appropriate response by the nurse? *(657)*
    1. "When you are using the ring, you will need to keep track of your periods and call if you miss one."
    2. "It is uncommon to miss a period while using the ring, but you will need to be seen by a healthcare provider if this happens."
    3. "Since missing one period is not uncommon, continue on the same cycle, but if two consecutive periods are missed a pregnancy test is needed."
    4. "Missing a period is not a concern, you may also experience spotting for two or more cycles which is also normal."

NCLEX item type: multiple response
Cognitive skill: application

15. Which information does the nurse include when teaching a patient about the use of the norelgestromin-ethinyl estradiol transdermal system (Ortho Evra)? *(Select all that apply.)* *(655)*
    1. "A new patch should be applied on the same day of the week."
    2. "Contraceptive therapy should be discontinued if pregnancy is confirmed."
    3. "Fold the used patch on itself and flush it down the toilet."
    4. "If the patch is detached for less than 24 hours, apply a new patch to the same location."
    5. "Report serious adverse effects such as severe headache, dizziness, blurred vision, and leg pain as soon as possible."

Copyright © 2023 by Elsevier, Inc. All rights reserved.

Scenario #2: A 78-year-old patient admitted to the hospital after a fall sustained a fractured femur. The patient had the fracture surgically repaired and subsequently diagnoses with osteoporosis. Their history is remarkable for diabetes mellitus, hypertension, depression, arthritis and atrial fibrillation.

Objective: Discuss osteoporosis and its risk factors as well as preventive measures and the pharmacologic treatment used.
NCLEX item type: multiple choice
Cognitive skill: interpret
16. A nurse educated the patient in scenario #2 about osteoporosis. The nurse knows further teaching is needed after the patient makes which statement? *(659)*
    1. "So you are saying that with this diagnosis of osteoporosis I will have fragile bones."
    2. "As I understand it, since I am also taking an anticoagulant that it can make the osteoporosis worse."
    3. "If I take more calcium and vitamin D and do strengthening exercises, I can preserve bone strength."
    4. "If I stop smoking and watch my alcohol intake to not exceed two drink daily, I can reverse this osteoporosis."
NCLEX item type: multiple response
Cognitive skill: compare
17. The nurse discussed the drugs used for treatment of osteoporosis with the patient in scenario #2. Which drugs will the nurse discuss? *(Select all that apply.)* *(660-661)*
    1. teriparatide
    2. denosumab
    3. ibandronate
    4. alfuzosin
    5. zoledronic acid
NCLEX item type: multiple choice
Cognitive skill: classify
18. The nurse recognized that the drug class bisphosphonates used for osteoporosis have which mechanism of action? *(660)*
    1. They directly affect the bone reabsorption that occurs by the osteoblasts.
    2. They decrease the rate of bone resorption by inhibiting bone resorption action of the osteoclasts.
    3. They indirectly affect the bone formation rate by enhancing the bone remodeling effect of the osteoblasts.
    4. They cause the calcium and vitamin D in the diet to directly impact the amount of bone laid down for rebuilding.

Objective: Describe pharmacologic treatments of benign prostatic hyperplasia.
NCLEX item type: grid/matrix
Cognitive skill: recognize cues
19. A nurse is describing the difference between the symptoms of obstructive and irritative benign prostatic hyperplasia (BPH) to a patient. Indicate with an 'X' the symptoms associated with obstructive and irritative BPH*(662)*

	Obstructive BPH	Irritative BPH
Decreased or interrupted urine stream		
Urge incontinence		
Reduced urine flow		
Sensation of incomplete bladder emptying		
Increased frequency		
Sudden urinary urgency		
Double voiding		

NCLEX item type: multiple choice
Cognitive skill: relate
20. When teaching a patient about dutasteride (Avodart) therapy for BPH, which statement does the nurse include? *(664)*
    1. "Dutasteride is also used to treat male pattern baldness."
    2. "Dutasteride will cause an increase in serum prostate-specific antigen (PSA) levels."
    3. "If there is no improvement of symptoms after 2 weeks of treatment, the dutasteride will be discontinued."
    4. "Men treated with dutasteride should not donate blood until at least 6 months after stopping therapy."
NCLEX item type: multiple choice
Cognitive skill: contrast
21. The nurse reviewed the medications used for BPH. Which medication works by inhibiting 5-alpha reductase type 2? *(664)*
    1. finasteride
    2. tamsulosin
    3. dutasteride
    4. sildenafil

Copyright © 2023 by Elsevier, Inc. All rights reserved.

Objective: Describe the pharmacologic treatment of erectile dysfunction.

NCLEX item type: multiple choice
Cognitive skill: analyze

22. The nurse is teaching a patient about tadalafil (Cialis) therapy. Which statement made by the patient indicates teaching has been successful? *(666-667)*
    1. "This drug is an aphrodisiac."
    2. "If I develop chest pain, I will take nitroglycerin."
    3. "I can expect the medication to work within 30 minutes."
    4. "I will take this medication three times a day on a regular basis."

NCLEX item type: multiple choice
Cognitive skill: illustrate

23. The nurse educated a patient regarding sildenafil and asked the patient to teach back. Which statement made by the patient about sildenafil (Viagra) therapy indicates further teaching is needed? *(667-668)*
    1. "I know that Viagra can cause patients to develop glaucoma."
    2. "I know that I should not take nitroglycerin for any angina while I am on Viagra."
    3. "I understand that if I suddenly lose my vision, I need to report it immediately."
    4. "If I get an erection that lasts longer than 4 hours I will seek medical attention."

NCLEX item type: multiple response
Cognitive skill: application

24. The nurse is educating the patient on the common adverse effects to expect when taking avanafil (Stendra) to treat erectile dysfunction, and includes which statements in the teaching? *(Select all that apply.)* *(667-668)*
    1. "Seek medical attention right away if you develop a sudden loss of hearing."
    2. "You need to be careful with nitrates in your food as they will react with the avanafil."
    3. "If you get dizzy or develop low blood pressure, lie down and let the symptoms pass."
    4. "If you develop any headache or flushing in your face and neck, these symptoms tend to be self-limiting."
    5. "It has been reported that if you become color-blind to blue or green, call your prescriber to get a dosage adjustment."

Copyright © 2023 by Elsevier, Inc. All rights reserved.

Drugs Used to Treat Disorders of the Urinary System

Answer Key: Textbook page references are provided as a guide for answering these questions. A complete answer key is provided to your instructor.

MATCHING

Match the definition on the right with the key term on the left.

Key Term

1. _____ urgency
2. _____ pyelonephritis
3. _____ frequency
4. _____ prostatitis
5. _____ overflow incontinence
6. _____ nocturia
7. _____ incontinence

Definition

a. infection of the kidneys
b. waking during the night with the need to void
c. the need to void eight or more times daily
d. a compelling desire to urinate that is difficult to ignore
e. the inability to control urine from passing from the bladder
f. chronic urinary retention
g. infection of the prostate gland

REVIEW QUESTIONS

Scenario #1: A 52-year-old female patient came to the clinic with complaints of burning on urination and foul-smelling urine. She told the nurse that this happens about twice a year.

Discuss the adverse effects of the drugs used to treat disorders of the urinary tract.
NCLEX item type: multiple response
Cognitive skill: instructions
8. The nurse educated the patient in scenario #1 who had a prescription for a urinary infection. What are the important instructions the nurse will include regarding antimicrobial agents for urinary infections? (*Select all that apply.*) **(674)**
   1. "You should take the entire course of the medication and not discontinue the medication when symptoms improve."
   2. "There are only two antimicrobial agents that are used for urinary tract infections."
   3. "You need to be sure to take adequate fluids because this will help dilute the urine."
   4. "We can teach you Kegel exercises and bladder training as well as the need to respond to the urge to void."
   5. "To avoid future infections cotton underwear is recommended and void bubble baths."

NCLEX item type: multiple choice
Cognitive skill: compare
9. The nurse reviews the medications used for the treatment of urinary tract infections and understands that there a single-dose treatment agent known as what? **(675)**
   1. nitrofurantoin
   2. fosfomycin
   3. mirabegron
   4. oxybutynin

NCLEX item type: multiple choice
Cognitive skill: classify
10. The nurse educated the patient in scenario #1 on the various conditions of common urinary tract infections. Which ones did the nurse indicate? (*Select all that apply.*) **(671)**
   1. Vaginitis
   2. Cystitis
   3. Pyelonephritis
   4. Urethritis
   5. Prostatitis

Copyright © 2023 by Elsevier, Inc. All rights reserved.

NCLEX item type: multiple choice
Cognitive skill: compare
11. The nurse recognizes the antimicrobial agents are used for bladder infections. Which of the antimicrobial agents listed are used for urinary infections? *(Select all that apply.)* **(674-675)**
    1. cephalexin
    2. fosfomycin
    3. linezolid
    4. ciprofloxacin
    5. nitrofurantoin

Identify important nursing interventions associated with the drug therapy and treatment of diseases of the urinary system.
NCLEX item type: grid/matrix
Cognitive skill: evaluate cues
12. When patients are taking antibiotics for urinary tract infections the nurse needs to perform interventions associated with the drug therapy. Indicate with an 'X' which interventions are appropriate and which ones are of no value for urinary tract infections. **(674)**

	Appropriate nursing interventions	Interventions that are of no value for urinary infections
Recording baseline vital signs		
Instructing patient to limit fluid intake		
Recording voiding characteristics		
Instructing patient on Kegel exercises		
Assessing for existing GI complaints prior to therapy		
Applying a transdermal patch to intact skin		
Educating patient on taking entire course of medication		

NCLEX item type: multiple response
Cognitive skill: application
13. The nurse will assess the patient in scenario #1 to gather what baseline data? *(Select all that apply.)* **(671-672)**
    1. History of urinary tract symptoms
    2. Medication history
    3. Nutritional history
    4. History of current symptoms
    5. Obtain a urine sample for analysis

NCLEX item type: multiple response
Cognitive skill: compare
14. The nurse recognizes which patients are considered to have a urinary tract infection? *(Select all that apply.)* **(671)**
    1. Male with prostatitis
    2. Female with vaginitis
    3. Male with pyelonephritis
    4. Female diagnosed with cystitis
    5. 4-year-old male with urethritis

NCLEX item type: multiple choice
Cognitive skill: classify
15. A patient is experiencing burning, frequency, pain, and urgency associated with a urinary tract infection. The nurse expects the healthcare provider to prescribe which medication to treat these symptoms? **(680)**
    1. phenazopyridine hydrochloride (Pyridium)
    2. oxybutynin chloride (Ditropan XL)
    3. mirabegron (Myrbetriq)
    4. nitrofurantoin (Macrodantin)

NCLEX item type: multiple response
Cognitive skill: interpret
16. The nurse knows that an important component of patient education to increase compliance with medications is to determine if the patient can verbalize which points? *(Select all that apply.)* **(674)**
    1. The name of drug
    2. The dosage of the drug
    3. The correct identification of the specific pathogen
    4. The common and adverse effects of the drug
    5. The timing of administration of the drug

NCLEX item type: multiple response
Cognitive skill: application
17. What important health teachings should the nurse complete for the patient in scenario #1 who has been prescribed nitrofurantoin (Macrodantin)? *(Select all that apply.)* **(675-676)**
    1. The patient needs to drink plenty of fluids.
    2. The patient needs to return for urine culture when scheduled.
    3. The patient should be instructed on the importance of continuing the medication for the entire course of treatment.
    4. The nurse should discuss personal hygiene measures—wiping front to back in females, keeping perineal area clean.
    5. The nurse should discuss symptoms such as perineal itching or vaginal discharge, when they occur to wait several days to see if they will resolve on their own.

Copyright © 2023 by Elsevier, Inc. All rights reserved.

NCLEX item type: multiple choice
Cognitive skill: relate
18. The nurse educates the patient in scenario #1 about phenazopyridine hydrochloride (Pyridium) for the treatment urinary tract infections. Which statement by the nurse needs to be corrected? *(680)*
    1. "The drug Pyridium reduces the bladder spasms that you are having."
    2. "You should be aware that Pyridium causes the color of urine to become reddish-orange."
    3. "The way Pyridium works is that it produces a local anesthetic effect on the mucosa of the ureters and bladder."
    4. "Pyridium is most effective against gram-negative bacterial urinary tract infections."

Scenario #2: The nurse interviewed a patient who came to the clinic with complaints of leaking urine, even after voiding. The patient was diagnosed with overflow incontinence.

Identify the symptoms, treatment, and medication used for overactive bladder syndrome.
NCLEX item type: multiple response
Cognitive skill: application
19. Which statements does the nurse include when teaching the patient in scenario #2 about overactive bladder syndrome? *(Select all that apply.) (677)*
    1. "You should avoid caffeine."
    2. "Overactive bladder syndrome cannot be cured."
    3. "A chronic infection is the cause of overactive bladder syndrome."
    4. "The first line of pharmacologic treatment of overactive bladder syndrome is anticholinergic agents."
    5. "The goals of therapy for overactive bladder syndrome are to decrease frequency by increasing voided volume, decreasing urgency, and reducing incidents of urinary urge incontinence."

NCLEX item type: cloze
Cognitive skill: recognize cues
20. **Choose the most likely options for the information missing from the statements below by selecting from the list of options provided.**
The nurse recognized the drugs _____1_____ and _____1_____ that are included in the anticholinergic agents used for_____2_____. *(677-678)*

Option 1	Option 2
mirabegron (Myrbetriq)	Bladder training
fosfomycin (Monurol)	Urinary tract infections
oxybutynin (Ditropan)	Overactive bladder syndrome
trospium (Sanctura)	Testing urine samples

NCLEX item type: multiple choice
Cognitive skill: compare
21. The nurse reviews the three primary symptoms of overactive bladder syndrome with the patient in scenario #2. Which symptoms does the nurse include in the discussion? *(676)*
    1. Frequency, urinary infections, and urinary incontinence
    2. Urgency, nocturia, and urge incontinence
    3. Nocturia, frequency, and stress incontinence
    4. Frequency, urgency, and urinary incontinence

Copyright © 2023 by Elsevier, Inc. All rights reserved.

Drugs Used to Treat Glaucoma and Other Eye Disorders

chapter

42

Answer Key: Textbook page references are provided as a guide for answering these questions. A complete answer key is provided to your instructor.

MATCHING
Match the key term on the right with the definition on the left.

Definition

1. _____ runs radially from the pupillary margin to the iris periphery

2. _____ sudden increase in intraocular pressure (IOP) caused by an obstruction in the iridocorneal angle

3. _____ dilation of the pupils

4. _____ within the iris that encircles the pupil

5. _____ paralysis of the ciliary muscle

6. _____ contraction of the iris sphincter muscle

7. _____ develops insidiously and causes changes in the iridocorneal angle

Key Term

a. miosis
b. mydriasis
c. cycloplegia
d. sphincter muscle
e. open-angle glaucoma
f. closed-angle glaucoma
g. dilator muscle

REVIEW QUESTIONS

Scenario #1: A 63-year-old male patient comes into the clinic with complaints of pain and constant tearing in his right eye after a flag whipped around his head and caught his eye. He is diagnosed with a corneal abrasion.

Objective: Explain patient assessments needed for eye disorders.
NCLEX item type: multiple response
Cognitive skill: explain

8. The nurse explains to the patient in scenario #1 the need for an eye examination that will include which assessments? (*Select all that apply*.) (686)
   1. Vision screening with a Snellen chart
   2. Observe for eyelid edema
   3. Observe for nystagmus
   4. Determine whether contact lenses are worn
   5. Determine whether the tear ducts are blocked

NCLEX item type: multiple response
Cognitive skill: application

9. What education will the nurse include in the patient instructions for the patient in scenario #1 with an eye injury ? (*Select all that apply.*) (686)
   1. "When the cornea gets abraded, it is highly susceptible to infection."
   2. "This injury has involved part of the sclera, the white portion of the eyeball."
   3. "This injury will effect the ability of the eye to dilate properly."
   4. "Colorblindness may occur with injury to the cornea."
   5. "When the cornea is seriously injured the resulting scar is not transparent."

NCLEX item type: multiple choice
Cognitive skill: relate

10. One of the greatest challenges in the care of chronic eye disorders such as glaucoma is convincing the patient of what? (*686*)
   1. The need to wear an eye patch every night to prevent eye strain
   2. The importance of not taking any over-the-counter or herbal products
   3. The differences among cataracts, glaucoma, and macular degeneration
   4. The need for long-term treatment and adherence to the therapeutic regimen

Copyright © 2023 by Elsevier, Inc. All rights reserved.

NCLEX item type: multiple
Cognitive skill: evaluate cues

11. The nurse is teaching the patient in scenario #2 the assessments needed for patients with glaucoma. Which instruction by the nurse needs to be revised? *(687-688)*
    1. "You will need to avoid heavy lifting, and straining on stools to prevent an increase in IOP."
    2. "It is important that you take your medication as directed, to prevent blindness."
    3. "The proper way to wipe your eyes is from the outside edges to the inner canthus."
    4. "You will be taught how to administers eye drops so you do not get an infection."

NCLEX item type: multiple choice
Cognitive skill: compare

12. The nurse explains to the patient in scenario #2 that when they have their IOP measured, it determines the eye's what? *(685)*
    1. Tear duct capacity
    2. Resistance from the ciliary bodies
    3. Amount of intraocular pressure, resulting from excess aqueous humor
    4. Ability to contract and relax the dilator muscle

NCLEX item type: drop and drag
Cognitive skill: recognize cues

13. The nurse reviewed the disorders of the eye and recognized the treatment used for each. *((693, 697-698))*

Indicate with an arrow which eye disorder uses which eye medication.

Macular degeneration	Ophthalmic antibiotics
Examine the interior of the eye, measure refraction	Artificial tears
Glaucoma	Rho kinase inhibitors
Lubrication of the eyes	Diagnostic agents
Fitting hard contacts	Vascular endothelial growth factor antagonists
Superficial eye infections	Anticholinergic agents

Scenario #2: A patient newly diagnosed with glaucoma come in to the clinic to get further instruction on how to manage the condition.

Objective: Identify patient teaching needs for patients with glaucoma.

NCLEX item type: multiple response
Cognitive skill: ordering

14. The nurse instructed the patient in scenario #2 on how to instill eye drops for treatment of glaucoma. List in the correct order how to instill eyedrops or eye ointment. *(688)*
    1. _____ Perform hand hygiene
    2. _____ Approach the eye from below
    3. _____ Apply gentle pressure using a clean tissue to the inner canthus of the eyelid
    4. _____ Instruct the patient to look up, and instill drops or squeeze ointment into the conjunctival sac
    5. _____ Expose the lower conjunctival sac by applying gentle traction

NCLEX item type: multiple response
Cognitive skill: application

15. Which statements does the nurse include when teaching a patient about health promotion after eye surgery? *(Select all that apply.)* *(687-688)*
    1. "Some medications may reduce visual acuity, keep in mind your safety."
    2. "Report any persistent redness or drainage from the eyes."
    3. "Cough at least 10 times every hour."
    4. "Report any pain not relieved by prescribed medications."
    5. "Use aseptic technique when instilling eye medications."

NCLEX item type: multiple choice
Cognitive skill: evaluate

16. The nurse was discussing the difference between open-angle glaucoma and closed-angle glaucoma with the patient in scenario #2 who was newly diagnosed with glaucoma. Which statement by the patient indicates more teaching is needed? *(685)*
    1. "Closed-angle glaucoma is the one that suddenly develops."
    2. "Open-angle glaucoma is the kind that develops slowly."
    3. "Glaucoma can be cured by taking eyedrops for 2 weeks."
    4. "Glaucoma is an eye disorder that develops because the pressure inside your eyeball is too high."

Copyright © 2023 by Elsevier, Inc. All rights reserved.

Objective: Discuss the medications used in the management of open-angle glaucoma.

NCLEX item type: multiple choice
Cognitive skill: contrast
17. The nurse reviews the mechanism of action for carbonic anhydrase inhibitors used for glaucoma. Which statement by the nurse is correct? *(688-689)*
    1. "Carbonic anhydrase inhibitors dilate the pupil and cause paralysis of the ciliary muscle."
    2. "Carbonic anhydrase inhibitors relax the ciliary muscle, and dilate the pupil."
    3. "Carbonic anhydrase inhibitors reduce the IOP by increasing the outflow of aqueous humor"
    4. "rbonic anhydrase inhibitors decrease the production of aqueous humor, thus lowering IOP."

NCLEX item type: multiple response
Cognitive skill: application
18. The nurse teaching the patient in scenario #2 about the use of the anticholinergic agent atropine sulfate and cautioned the patient to be aware of systemic adverse effects. Which effects need to be reported to the healthcare provider? *(Select all that apply.)* *(693)*
    1. Tachycardia
    2. Diarrhea
    3. Blurred vision
    4. Urinary retention
    5. Dry mouth

NCLEX item type: multiple choice
Cognitive skill: evaluate outcomes
19. The nurse recognized beta-adrenergic blocking agents work by which mechanism of action when given for the treatment of glaucoma? *(691)*
    1. By reducing the production of aqueous humor
    2. By causing pupil dilation, increased outflow of aqueous humor, and vasoconstriction
    3. By increasing the outflow of aqueous humor
    4. By increasing the trabecular meshwork outflow

Copyright © 2023 by Elsevier, Inc. All rights reserved.

Drugs Used to Treat Cancer

chapter

43

Answer Key: Textbook page references are provided as a guide for answering these questions. A complete answer key is provided to your instructor.

MATCHING
Match the definition on the left with the term on the right.

Definition

1. _____ biologic therapies that include cytokines, monoclonal antibodies, growth factors, and vaccines

2. _____ chemotherapy that uses cell cycle–specific and cell cycle–nonspecific agents

3. _____ meaning new growth; can refer to benign or malignant cells

4. _____ abnormal cell growth that invades surrounding tissues and develops growths in other tissues distant to the site of origin

5. _____ agents that help reduce the toxicity of chemotherapeutic agents to normal cells

6. _____ ancer cells that metastasize to other organs of the body

Term

a. metastases
b. malignant
c. targeted anticancer agents
d. chemoprotective agents
e. neoplastic disease
f. combination therapy

REVIEW QUESTIONS

Scenario #1: A 48-year-old woman, mother of three, was newly diagnosed with breast cancer and was very distraught in the outpatient clinic when she came for her first chemotherapy treatment.

Objective: Discuss the goals of chemotherapy.
NCLEX item type: multiple response
Cognitive skill: application

7. The nurse explained to the patient in scenario #1 the goals of chemotherapy. Which goals does the nurse include in the discussion? *(Select all that apply.)* *(701-702)*
   1. A goal for chemotherapy is to control the growth of the cancer cells
   2. A goal for chemotherapy is long-term survival or a cure
   3. A goal for chemotherapy is to use phase-nonspecific chemotherapy agents exclusively
   4. A goal of chemotherapy is to administer the drugs when new pathways of tumor cell metabolism are discovered
   5. A goal of chemotherapy is to give doses large enough to kill the cancer cells but small enough for normal cells to live

NCLEX item type: multiple choice
Cognitive skill: evaluate

8. After educating the patient in scenario #1 about the best timing for giving chemotherapy, the nurse knows that which statement by the patient would indicate further teaching is needed? *(701-702,709)*
   1. "I know that the overall goal of chemotherapy in general is to give enough drug to kill the cancer without too much damage to the normal cells."
   2. "I understand it is important to deliver the chemotherapy at precise intervals to impact the cancer cells' growth cycle."
   3. "I can prevent complications from the chemotherapy through proper diet and hygiene."
   4. "I understand that when I am on chemotherapy, I can have fresh flowers as long as I do not touch them and I can eat fresh vegetables that I wash thoroughly."

Copyright © 2023 by Elsevier, Inc. All rights reserved.

NCLEX item type: multiple response
Cognitive skill: relate

9. For the patient and family to manage the chemotherapy treatment regimen, an understanding of which points needs to be stressed by the nurse? *(Select all that apply.)* *(710)*
   1. Name of the drug
   2. Right documentation
   3. Common and serious adverse effects
   4. Time of administration
   5. Dosage and route of the drug

NCLEX item type: multiple response
Cognitive skill: application

10. The nurse explains to the patient in scenario #1 that the treatment of cancer often requires multiple different approaches, which may include what modalities? *(Select all that apply.)* *(700)*
    1. Surgery
    2. Radiation
    3. Biologic therapies
    4. Targeted drug therapy
    5. Phlebotomy

Objective: Describe the role of targeted anticancer agents in treating cancer.

NCLEX item type: multiple response
Cognitive skill: explain

11. The nurse discussed with the patient in scenario #1 the choice of chemotherapeutic agents used to help fight cancer depend on certain characteristic of the cancer. Which characteristics does the nurse explain to the patient? *(Select all that apply.)* *(702)*
    1. The size of the tumor
    2. The type of tumor cell
    3. The potency of the agent
    4. The rate of growth of the cancer
    5. The frequency of the agents' administration

NCLEX item type: multiple choice
Cognitive skill: compare

12. The nurse reviewed the use of targeted anticancer agents in the treatment of cancer with the patient in scenario #1. Which statement by the nurse needs to be corrected? *(704)*
    1. "The targeted anticancer agents are designed to trigger the recovery of the bone marrow cells."
    2. "Biologic therapies also known as targeted anticancer agents are noncytotoxic drugs that target key pathways of cancer cells."
    3. "These targeted anticancer agents include cytokines, monoclonal antibodies, growth factors and vaccines."
    4. "Targeted agents are not associated with severe toxicities common with cytotoxic therapy, but allergic reactions are common."

NCLEX item type: grid/matrix
Cognitive skill: recognize cues

13. The nurse classified the drugs considered part of the traditional major groups of chemotherapeutic agents. Indicate with an 'X' the chemotherapy agents considered traditional and the agents that are the newer group of agents. *(702-704)*

	Traditional agents	**Newer agents**
Hormones		
Antimetabolites		
Alkylating agents		
Checkpoint inhibitors		
Mitotic inhibitors		
Topoisomerase inhibitors		
Antineoplastic antibodies		
Tyrosine kinase inhibitors		
Biologic therapies		

NCLEX item type: cloze
Cognitive skill: evaluate cues

Choose the most likely options for the information missing from the statements below by selecting from the list of options provided.

14. The nurse reviewed the chemotherapy agents that are _____1_____ or _____1_____ and identified them as _____2_____ and _____2_____. *(704)*

Option 1	Option 2
Targeted anticancer agents	Cytokines
Traditional agents	Cholinesterase inhibitors
Biologic therapies	Alkylating agents
Checkpoint inhibitors	Growth factors

Copyright © 2023 by Elsevier, Inc. All rights reserved.

Scenario #2: The nurse taking care of a patient with lymphoma administered ordered treatments and assesses the patient for anticipated and adverse effects.

Objective: Identify how chemoprotective agents are used in treating cancer.
NCLEX item type: multiple choice
Cognitive skill: compare
15. The nurse administered a chemoprotective agent for the patient in scenario #2 used to treat cancer because of what effect? *(704)*
    1. Chemoprotective agents stimulate red blood cell production.
    2. Chemoprotective agents target the cancer cells specifically.
    3. Chemoprotective agents trigger the recovery of bone marrow cells.
    4. Chemoprotective agents reduce the toxic effects of the chemotherapy agents on normal cells.
NCLEX item type: multiple response
Cognitive skill: classify
16. The nurse reviewed the medications used as chemoprotective agents. Which drugs are part of this classification? *(Select all that apply.)* *(705)*
    1. sargramostim (Leukine)
    2. mesna (Mesnex)
    3. dexrazoxane (Totect)
    4. amifostine (Ethyol)
    5. filgrastim (Neupogen)
NCLEX item type: multiple response
Cognitive skill: application
17. The nurse is administering a chemotherapeutic agent to the patient in scenario #2 and knows which precautions must be observed for safe handling of these agents? *(Select all that apply.)* *(704)*
    1. Prevent any inhalation of aerosols.
    2. Carefully mix the agents in the med room.
    3. Prevent contamination of body fluids.
    4. Follow proper protocol for safe disposal of agents.
    5. Prevent any drug absorption through the skin.

Objective: Discuss bone marrow stimulants and their effect and use.
NCLEX item type: multiple response
Cognitive skill: application
18. The nurse teaching the patient in scenario #2 what the bone marrow stimulants do in the treatment of cancer. Which statement by the nurse will be included in the discussion? *(704)*
    1. They induce anemia.
    2. They stimulate the resting phase of the cell.
    3. They trigger an increase of killer T cells.
    4. They trigger the recovery of bone marrow cells.

NCLEX item type: multiple response
Cognitive skill: compare
19. The nurse anticipates the use of which medication to treat a patient with chemotherapy-induced anemia by stimulating the production of RBCs? *(705)*
    1. sargramostim (Leukine)
    2. glucarpidase (Voraxaze)
    3. epoetin alfa (Epogen)
    4. filgrastim (Neupogen)
NCLEX item type: multiple response
Cognitive skill: compare
20. The nurse orienting to an oncology unit learned about bone marrow stimulants. Which patient situations are bone marrow stimulants appropriate? *(Select all that apply.)* *(704)*
    1. For patients being treated for leukemia
    2. When patients are undergoing lymphoma therapy
    3. For those patients having bone marrow transplantation
    4. For patients to control cell membrane receptor response
    5. For patients to reduce the toxic effects of chemotherapy

Objective: Describe the nursing assessments and interventions needed to help alleviate the adverse effects of chemotherapy.
NCLEX item type: multiple response
Cognitive skill: take action
21. What are the baseline assessments the nurse will obtain for the patient in scenario #2 that are needed during the initiation of cancer therapy? *(Select all that apply.)* *(704,706)*
    1. Determine the exposure to tobacco and tobacco smoke.
    2. Identify the usual eating and elimination patterns.
    3. Ask about the understanding the patient has of the diagnosis.
    4. Review the medication history for any drugs that may have caused cancer.
    5. Ask about a history of viral disease that may have caused cancer.
NCLEX item type: multiple response
Cognitive skill: application
22. The nurse will monitor the patient in scenario #2 for adverse effects from chemotherapy. Which adverse effects can the nurse expect to find? *(Select all that apply.)* *(706)*
    1. Stomatitis (mucositis)
    2. Alopecia
    3. Heat intolerance
    4. Changes in bowel patterns
    5. Nausea and vomiting

Copyright © 2023 by Elsevier, Inc. All rights reserved.

NCLEX item type: multiple choice
Cognitive skill: generate solutions
23. A patient has severe lesions in their mouth as an adverse effect of chemotherapy. When does the nurse suggest the patient perform oral hygiene measures using prescribed local anesthetic and antimicrobial solutions? *(707-708)*
   1. After each meal
   2. Once every 8 hours
   3. Hourly while the patient is awake
   4. The morning when the patient awakens and before bed

Copyright © 2023 by Elsevier, Inc. All rights reserved.

Drugs Used to Treat the Musculoskeletal System

Answer Key: Textbook page references are provided as a guide for answering these questions. A complete answer key is provided to your instructor.

MATCHING

Match the definition on the right to the key term on the left.

Key Term

1. _____ cerebral palsy
2. _____ multiple sclerosis
3. _____ neuromuscular blocking agents
4. _____ hypercapnia
5. _____ spasticity
6. _____ muscle spasms
7. _____ gout

Definition

a. an upper motor neuron disorder characterized by muscle hypertonicity and involuntary jerks
b. caused by an injury or birth defect, characterized by exaggerated reflexes, abnormal posture, involuntary movements, and difficulty walking
c. elevated carbon dioxide levels causing tachycardia, hypotension, and cyanosis
d. sudden alternating contractions and relaxations or sustained contractions of muscle
e. a common and treatable form of inflammatory arthritis
f. an autoimmune disease affecting the brain and spinal cord
g. caused by an embolism, thrombosis, or ruptured aneurysm; characteristics include a sudden onset of vertigo, aphasia, and dysarthria, along with hemiplegia

REVIEW QUESTIONS

Scenario #1: A 35-year-old patient with cerebral palsy came into the outpatient clinic scheduled to have the baclofen pump refilled.

Objective: Describe the therapeutic effect of centrally acting skeletal muscle relaxants on the central nervous system and the common and serious adverse effects.

NCLEX item type: multiple choice
Cognitive skill: compare

8. The nurse reviewed the mechanism of action for the centrally acting skeletal muscle relaxants. Which action does the nurse recognize as how these drugs work? *(715)*
   1. They directly affect the muscles.
   2. They cause CNS depression.
   3. They affect nerve conduction.
   4. They cause the neuromuscular junctions to be desensitized to stimuli.

NCLEX item type: multiple response
Cognitive skill: compare

9. The nurse will check for common adverse effects related to the baclofen pump the patient in scenario #1 and specifically which symptoms? *(Select all that apply.)* *(717)*
   1. Drowsiness
   2. Fatigue
   3. Headache
   4. Back pain
   5. Dizziness

Copyright © 2023 by Elsevier, Inc. All rights reserved.

NCLEX item type: multiple response
Cognitive skill: evaluate cues

10. The nurse instructed the patient in scenario #1 about centrally acting skeletal muscle relaxants. Which statement by the nurse will be included in the teaching? *(Select all that apply.)* *(715,717)*
    1. "These drugs produce sedation in patients receiving them, so you need to be careful."
    2. "The medication you are on has a direct effect on the neuromuscular junction, causing relaxation of the muscles."
    3. "The drug baclofen produces a therapeutic effect by depressing the central nervous system."
    4. "These drugs will relieve muscle spasms associated with acute, painful musculoskeletal conditions."
    5. "These muscle relaxants are the agents of choice for the treatment of muscle spasticity associated with cerebral or spinal cord disease."

NCLEX item type: multiple response
Cognitive skill: application

11. The nurse reviewing laboratory results to determine if the patient on the centrally acting skeletal muscle relaxant chlorzoxazone (Lorzone) was exhibiting any hepatotoxicity. Which laboratory results would be important to monitor? *(Select all that apply.)* *(716)*
    1. ALP
    2. WBC
    3. RBC
    4. AST
    5. ALT

NCLEX item type: cloze
Cognitive skill: recognize cues

Choose the most likely options for the information missing from the statements below by selecting from the list of options provided.

12. The nurse needed to administer _____1_____ to the patient with acute back spasms, and recognized _____2_____ and _____2_____ as those drugs belonging to that class. *(715-716)*

Option 1	Option 2
Neuromuscular blocking agent	allopurinol (Zyloprim)
Central acting skeletal muscle relaxant	carisoprodol (Soma)
Xanthine oxidase inhibitors	metaxalone (Skelaxin)
Direct acting skeletal muscle relaxant	dantrolene (Dantrium)

NCLEX item type: multiple choice
Cognitive skill: interpret

13. Which statement by a patient taking dantrolene (Dantrium) for treatment of muscle spasticity of stroke syndrome indicates that more patient education is needed by the nurse? *(718)*
    1. "I will avoid exposure to the sun, but I can still use a tanning lamp."
    2. "I will notify my healthcare provider if my skin turns yellow."
    3. "I know that it might take up to a week for me to see any response to this drug."
    4. "If I develop adverse effects from this medication, I will not discontinue treatment until I notify my healthcare provider."

Objective: Describe the physiologic effects of neuromuscular blocking agents and the common and serious adverse effects.

NCLEX item type: multiple response
Cognitive skill: application

14. The nurse reviewed the patient scenarios when it would be appropriate to use neuromuscular blocking agents. Which examples are appropriate for use of these agents? *(Select all that apply.)* *(718)*
    1. When patients have tetanus
    2. When patients develop nystagmus
    3. During the administration of general anesthesia
    4. When intubating patients and preventing laryngospasm
    5. During the administration of electroshock therapy to prevent muscular activity

NCLEX item type: multiple choice
Cognitive skill: comprehension

15. Why would patients with myasthenia gravis, spinal cord injuries, or multiple sclerosis need to be carefully identified by an anesthetist prior to administration of neuromuscular blocking agents? *(719)*
    1. Postoperatively, these patients will experience respiratory depression for a prolonged period.
    2. These patients will develop the adverse effect of histamine release much faster than other patients.
    3. These patients will require larger doses of the agents to get the same effect as other patients.
    4. These patients need careful adjustments in dosages to assess their ability to tolerate the agents.

Copyright © 2023 by Elsevier, Inc. All rights reserved.

NCLEX item type: extended multiple response
Cognitive skill: recognize cues

16. A patient who has returned from abdominal surgery reports pain. The patient had received a neuromuscular blocking agent as part of the anesthesia for the surgery. What assessments and equipment are essential for the nurse to obtain before administering the prescribed analgesic? (*Select all that apply.*) **(718-719)**
    1. Respirations
    2. History for spinal cord injury
    3. Oxygen equipment
    4. Laboratory results for CBC and electrolytes
    5. Estimated time of discharge
    6. Suction equipment
    7. Patient controlled analgesic (PCA) pump
    8. Antidotes for neuromuscular blocking agents
    9. Temperature

NCLEX item type: multiple choice
Cognitive skill: compare

17. The nurse needs to observe for the common and serious adverse effects of neuromuscular blocking agents after patients receive them during surgery. Which effects need to be reported? (*Select all that apply.*) **(719)**
    1. Vital signs change from hypotension to hypertension
    3. Respiratory distress, diminished cough and inability to swallow
    4. Muscle paralysis that effects the eyelids
    5. Pain in the neck, upper back, and in the abdominal muscles

Scenario #2: A patient newly diagnosed with gout came to the clinic for further evaluation of gout management.

Objective: Identify the therapeutic response and the common and serious adverse effects from gout medications.

NCLEX item type: multiple choice
Cognitive skill: interpret

18. The nurse reviews the primary therapeutic outcome of colchicine therapy with the patient in scenario #2. Which outcome will be discussed? **(720)**
    1. Dissolve uric acid crystals
    2. Inhibit the production of uric acid
    3. Decrease the amount of uric acid in the blood or urine
    4. Eliminate joint pain secondary to acute gout attack

NCLEX item type: multiple choice
Cognitive skill: evaluate

19. The nurse has provided patient teaching for probenecid therapy. Which statement by the patient indicates that more teaching is needed? **(721)**
    1. "This drug works on the tissues of my great toe, where I usually get the gout, to get rid of the problem."
    2. "I can expect that the incidence of gout attacks may increase for the first few months of therapy with this drug."
    3. "I will tell my healthcare provider if I develop vomiting that looks like coffee grounds."
    4. "If I develop a rash, I will tell my healthcare provider because this most likely means that I have an allergy to this drug."

NCLEX item type: multiple choice
Cognitive skill: evaluate

20. After completing the education for the patient in scenario #2 on the use of colchicine, the nurse will need to provide further education when the patient makes which statement? **(720)**
    1. "I need to take this to prevent an attack of gout."
    2. "My joint swelling will subside within 12 hours."
    3. "It will take from 48 to 72 hours before I will get any pain relief."
    4. "I know I can take a dose every 3 days to prevent an attack of gout."

NCLEX item type: grid/matrix
Cognitive skill: evaluate outcomes

21. The nurse compared the uses for the gout agents colchicine, probenecid and xanthine oxidase inhibitors. Indicate with an arrow the effects each agent has. **(720-722)**

Gout agents	Uses for gout agents
colchicine	Treats primary hyperuricemia because it inhibits production of uric acid
febuxostat	Prevents and treats acute gout flares, relieving joint pain and swelling
probenecid	Chronic management of hyperuricemia
allopurinol	Enhances excretion of uric acid, not effective for acute gout attacks and not an analgesic

Copyright © 2023 by Elsevier, Inc. All rights reserved.

Antimicrobial Agents

Answer Key: Textbook page references are provided as a guide for answering these questions. A complete answer key is provided to your instructor.

MATCHING
Match the definition on the left with the term on the right.

Definition

1. _____ examples include: *Acinetobacter spp., Providencia spp., Escherichia coli,* and *Klebsiella spp.*

2. _____ damage to the eighth cranial nerve, causing dizziness, tinnitus, and hearing loss

3. _____ microorganisms that are toxic to patients

4. _____ examples include: *Staphylococcus aureus, S. epidermidis, Streptococcus pyogenes,* and *S. pneumoniae*

5. _____ antimicrobial therapy given to patients at risk for developing infections

6. _____ damage to the kidney, causing increased creatinine and BUN, and decreased urine output

7. _____ reduced circulating prothrombin, with and without bleeding

Term

a. pathogenic
b. prophylactic antibiotics
c. nephrotoxicity
d. ototoxicity
e. hypoprothrombinemia
f. Gram-negative microorganisms
g. Gram-positive microorganisms

REVIEW QUESTIONS

Scenario #1: An 89-year-old patient was admitted to the hospital with urosepsis. The patient has a history of diabetes, hypertension, hypothyroidism, depression, functional decline, and gastroesophageal reflux disease (GERD).

Objective: Explain the major actions and effects of classes of drugs used to treat infectious diseases.
NCLEX item type: multiple choice
Cognitive skill: compare
8. The nurse reviewed the antibiotics from the drug class macrolides and recognizes that they have which action on bacteria? *(738)*
   1. They prevent the bacteria from making folic acid.
   2. They inhibit the ability of the bacteria to synthesize protein.
   3. They inhibit the cell wall synthesis in bacteria.
   4. They prevent the replication of bacterial DNA.

NCLEX item type: multiple response
Cognitive skill: application
9. The nurse anticipates that the patient in scenario #1 may be started on an aminoglycoside, which can also be used to treat what other conditions? *(Select all that apply.)* *(729)*
   1. Wound infections
   2. Latent tuberculosis
   3. Viral infections
   4. Life-threatening septicemia
   5. Gram-negative bacteria causing meningitis

NCLEX item type: multiple choice
Cognitive skill: contrast
10. The patient in scenario #1 was started on doripenem an antimicrobial agent from the drug class carbapenems. The nurse knows this drug class will act on bacteria by what mechanism of action? *(730)*
   1. Carbapenems inhibit cell membrane synthesis.
   2. Carbapenems prevent bacteria from making folic acid.
   3. Carbapenems inhibit bacterial cell wall synthesis.
   4. Carbapenems prevent the replication of bacterial DNA.

Copyright © 2023 by Elsevier, Inc. All rights reserved.

NCLEX item type: extended multiple response
Cognitive skill: recognize cues

11. The nurse asked a student nurse to identify the class of antibiotics that inhibit protein synthesis in bacterial cells as their mechanism of action. Which classes does the student identify? (*Select all that apply.*) *(729,738-739,746,748)*
    1. Quinolones
    2. Streptogramins
    3. Macrolides
    4. Carbapenems
    5. Tetracyclines
    6. Aminoglycosides
    7. Penicillins
    8. Sulfonamides

NCLEX item type: multiple choice
Cognitive skill: compare

12. The nurse administered penicillin to a patient with an infection and remembered there was a class of antibiotics that are chemically related penicillins and act by inhibiting cell wall synthesis. Which drug class does this represent? *(732)*
    1. Quinolones
    2. Macrolides
    3. Streptogramins
    4. Cephalosporins

NCLEX item type: multiple choice
Cognitive skill: explain

13. The patient in scenario #1 mentioned to the nurse that they were allergic to levofloxacin a quinolone, and asked the nurse to explain how that drug works. Which statement by the nurse describes the mechanism of action of the quinolones? *(743-744)*
    1. "Bacteria have cell walls and the quinolones inhibit the ability of the bacteria to make a cell wall."
    2. "The quinolones are a class of antibiotics that work by preventing the replication of bacterial DNA."
    3. "The quinolones work by inhibiting the ability of the bacteria to synthesis proteins that the bacteria needs."
    4. "Quinolones work by inhibiting the bacteria's ability to make folic acid."

NCLEX item type: multiple choice
Cognitive skill: classify

14. The nurse recognizes the class of antimicrobials reserved for serious or life-threatening infections that are vancomycin-resistant such as VRE, and act by inhibiting protein synthesis in bacterial cells are called what? *(746)*
    1. Carbapenems
    2. Streptogramins
    3. Quinolones
    4. Cephalosporins

NCLEX item type: cloze
Cognitive skill: recognize cues

Choose the most likely options for the information missing from the statements below by selecting from the list of options provided.

15. The nurse administered ertapenem an antimicrobial effective against ____1_____and _____1_____, and knows its mechanism of action is by inhibiting _____2_____. *(731)*

Option 1	Option 2
Anaerobic bacteria	Key metabolic pathways needed for bacterial growth
Fungal infections	Bacterial cell wall synthesis
Aerobic bacteria	Bacterial biosynthesis of folic acid
Viral infections	Protein synthesis in bacteria

Objective: Describe the signs and symptoms of the common adverse effects of antimicrobial therapy.

NCLEX item type: multiple response
Cognitive skill: recognize cues

16. The patient in scenario #1 who was started on doripenem a carbapenem, asks the nurse about common adverse effects associated with antimicrobial therapy. Which symptoms are considered the 'big three' adverse effects of antimicrobial therapy that the nurse mentions? (*Select all that apply.*) *(727)*
    1. Nausea
    2. Vomiting
    3. Allergies
    4. Constipation
    5. Diarrhea

NCLEX item type: multiple choice
Cognitive skill: compare

17. The patient in the scenario #1 was switched to cefuroxime after developing an allergy to the other antibiotic. Which medication prescribed for another clinical condition did the nurse notice was contraindicated with cefuroxime because of known drug interactions and requires notifying the prescriber? *(735)*
    1. metformin (Glucophage)
    2. atenolol (Tenormin)
    3. famotidine (Pepcid)
    4. levothyroxine (Synthroid)

NCLEX item type: multiple response
Cognitive skill: take action

18. Prior to administration of a carbapenem to the patient in scenario #1, what premedication assessments should the nurse perform? (*Select all that apply.*) *(732)*
    1. Check hydration status.
    2. Check vital signs.
    3. Assess basic mental status.
    4. Check any allergies specifically to penicillin and cephalosporins.
    5. Determine that the organism being treated is *Candida albicans*.

Copyright © 2023 by Elsevier, Inc. All rights reserved.

NCLEX item type: multiple choice
Cognitive skill: comprehension
19. The nurse was performing a premedication assessment before therapy with cephalosporins on a patient. Which condition observed in the patient would indicate the drug should be held and the healthcare provider notified? *(733)*
    1. Exophthalmos
    2. Oral candidiasis
    3. Onychomycosis of the toenail
    4. Low urine output and concentrated urine

Scenario #2: A patient admitted to the hospital with fever, productive cough and pain on inspiration was diagnosed with pneumonia. After sputum cultures were obtained the patient was started on an antibiotic.

Objective: Describe the nursing assessments and interventions for the common adverse effects associated with antimicrobial agents: allergic reaction, nephrotoxicity, ototoxicity, and hepatotoxicity.

NCLEX item type: multiple response
Cognitive skill: application
20. The assessment data that the nurse will monitor for the patient in scenario #2 who has now been receiving piperacillin/tazobactam (Zosyn) for the pneumonia, include noting which signs and symptoms? *(Select all that apply.)* **(741)**
    1. Any photosensitivity
    2. Any allergic reactions
    3. When the last vaccination for flu was given
    4. Changes in laboratory results (i.e., BUN and creatinine)
    5. Any symptoms that may indicate a secondary infection is developing

NCLEX item type: multiple response
Cognitive skill: evaluate outcomes
21. The nurse educated the patient in scenario #2 on the symptoms of hepatotoxicity to be monitored for after discharge from the hospital. Which statements by the nurse are included in the instructions? *(Select all that apply.)* **(727-728)**
    1. "One of the ways we check for hepatotoxicity is if you start to get anorexic and lose your appetite."
    2. "Sometimes your skin will turn yellow, we call this getting jaundice and it is a sign of hepatotoxicity."
    3. "When your laboratory values start to show an elevated creatinine, we get worried."
    4. "A symptom of hepatotoxicity is hepatomegaly which is an enlarged liver."
    5. "You may start to get episodes of nausea and vomiting which when that occurs in conjunction with other symptoms leads to hepatotoxicity."

NCLEX item type: multiple response
Cognitive skill: recognize cues
22. The nurse monitored the patient in scenario #2 for the severe adverse reaction of nephrotoxicity from antimicrobial therapy by which laboratory results? *(Select all that apply.)* **(727)**
    1. AST
    2. Creatinine
    3. WBC
    4. BUN
    5. Hgb

NCLEX item type: multiple choice
Cognitive skill: comprehension
23. The nurse was asked by a patient, "why is it essential to report the occurrence of severe diarrhea with antibiotic therapy?" Which response by the nurse accurately answers the question? **(727)**
    1. "Antibiotic therapy can indicate nephrotoxicity."
    2. "This may mean that the drug is not being absorbed any further."
    3. "When this happens it may indicate drug-induced pseudomembranous colitis."
    4. "An allergic response to the antibiotic has occurred."

NCLEX item type: multiple response
Cognitive skill: application
24. The nurse will monitor the patient in scenario #2 carefully for which signs and symptoms of a secondary infection? *(Select all that apply.)* **(727)**
    1. Anal lesions
    2. Severe diarrhea
    3. Phlebitis at the IV site
    4. Tinnitus and progressive hearing loss
    5. White patches in the oral cavity

NCLEX item type: multiple response
Cognitive skill: application
25. When administering an aminoglycoside such as tobramycin to a patient, what premedication assessment does the nurse perform? *(Select all that apply.)* **(730)**
    1. Determine any history of renal disease
    2. Assess for adequate hydration status related to any nausea and vomiting
    3. Determine if there is any symptoms of hearing loss
    4. Assess whether anesthesia was administered to the patient within the past 48–72 hours
    5. Determine any allergy to penicillin because patients allergic to penicillin are allergic to aminoglycosides

NCLEX item type: multiple choice
Cognitive skill: contrast
26. A patient who was being treated for cellulitis with an antibiotic returned to the clinic with complaints of his arm looking sunburnt and developing patches that itch after being outside. The nurse recognizes these symptoms as what adverse effect? **(728)**
    1. Blood dyscrasia
    2. Photosensitivity
    3. Nephrotoxicity
    4. Secondary infection

Copyright © 2023 by Elsevier, Inc. All rights reserved.

NCLEX item type: multiple choice
Cognitive skill: evaluate
27. After completing education on levofloxacin for a patient with a sinus infection, the nurse knows that more teaching is needed when the patient makes which statement? *(745-746)*
    1. "I know I need to call my provider if I start to get numbness and tingling in my legs."
    2. "If I develop a headache, I will just take some over-the-counter NSAIDs."
    3. "I know that my kidneys may be affected with this antibiotic, so I will report any decline in my urine output."
    4. "Since I am diabetic I know to check my blood sugar more frequently as this drug can cause hypoglycemia."

Objective: Discuss the primary uses for antibiotic agents, antitubercular agents, antifungal agents, and antiviral agents.
NCLEX item type: multiple choice
Cognitive skill: explain
28. After being treated with an antibiotic for several days the patient in scenario #1 developed oral thrush, from *Candida albicans*. The nurse explained to the patient the medication being used to treat this and how it works. Which statement by the nurse is correct? *(757)*
    1. "Antifungal agents work by inhibiting the bacteria's ability to synthesize folic acid."
    2. "Antifungal agents work by inhibiting DNA synthesis of the bacterial cells."
    3. "Antifungal agents disrupt the cell membrane of the fungal cells."
    4. "Antifungal agents interfere with the enzyme needed for cell wall generation."

NCLEX item type: multiple response
Cognitive skill: classify
29. The nurse explains to the patient in scenario #2 that antimicrobial agents can be classified according to the types of pathogenic organisms. Which organisms does the nurse mention? *(Select all that apply.) (725)*
    1. Pollen
    2. Fungus
    3. Cerumen
    4. Viruses
    5. Bacteria

NCLEX item type: multiple choice
Cognitive skill: comprehension
30. The nurse was assigned a patient who developed herpes simplex during the hospitalization and expects to find which medication ordered for this infection? *(764)*
    1. acyclovir (Zovirax)
    2. fluconazole (Diflucan)
    3. daptomycin (Cubicin)
    4. tigecycline (Tygacil)

NCLEX item type: multiple response
Cognitive skill: application
31. The nurse recognized that there are several types of infections that macrolides can be used for. Which types of infections does the nurse recognize? *(Select all that apply.) (738)*
    1. Respiratory
    2. Gastrointestinal tract
    3. Prophylactic before surgery
    4. Sexually transmitted infection
    5. Skin and soft-tissue infections

NCLEX item type: multiple response
Cognitive skill: application
32. A patient newly prescribed the cephalosporin Ceclor asked the nurse how they would know if they were experiencing an allergic reaction. What would be an appropriate response by the nurse? *(Select all that apply.) (727)*
    1. "Some allergic reactions can be fatal like anaphylaxis that causes laryngeal edema, dyspnea and shock."
    2. "Allergic reactions can occur within 30 minutes of administration or they could be delayed."
    3. "Nausea, vomiting, and diarrhea are the most common symptoms of an allergic reaction."
    4. "Trouble breathing, skin rashes, or facial edema may be symptoms of an allergic reaction."
    5. "Most of the time allergic reactions rarely occur with antibiotics."

NCLEX item type: multiple choice
Cognitive skill: evaluate
33. The nurse reviewed the effects of administering tetracyclines during pregnancy and early childhood and remembered they were not be given because they will cause what to occur? *(748)*
    1. Dental caries
    2. Tooth enamel staining
    3. An allergy to penicillin
    4. Bleeding gums

NCLEX item type: multiple choice
Cognitive skill: classify
34. The nurse preparing isoniazid and rifampin to be administered to a patient knows that these antibiotics are being given for the treatment of what? *(750,752)*
    1. Syphilis
    2. Trichinosis
    3. Tuberculosis
    4. Cellulitis

NCLEX item type: multiple response
Cognitive skill: application
35. The nurse had an order to administer the topical antifungal agent ketoconazole and knows it is used to treat which patient conditions? *(Select all that apply.) (758)*
    1. Herpes simplex
    2. Tinea pedis (athlete's foot)
    3. Candidiasis (thrush)
    4. Cutaneous candidiasis (diaper rash)
    5. Tinea corporis (ringworm)

Copyright © 2023 by Elsevier, Inc. All rights reserved.

Nutrition

Answer Key: Textbook page references are provided as a guide for answering these questions. A complete answer key is provided to your instructor.

MATCHING
Match the definition on the right with the key term on the left.

Key Term

1. _____ Dietary Reference Intakes (DRIs)
2. _____ Estimated Average Requirement (EAR)
3. _____ Recommended Dietary Allowances (RDAs)
4. _____ Adequate Intake (AI)
5. _____ Tolerable Upper Intake Level (UL)
6. _____ Estimated Energy Requirement (EER)
7. _____ marasmus
8. _____ kwashiorkor

Definition

a. the highest level of daily nutrient intake that is likely to pose no risk of adverse health effects
b. a list of average daily dietary intake level that meets the nutrient requirements of almost all healthy individuals in a group
c. the most common form of malnutrition in hospitalized patients
d. the average dietary energy intake that is predicted to maintain energy balance in healthy adults
e. provides quantitative estimates of nutrient intakes for planning and assessing diets
f. a protein deficiency that develops when little or no protein is in the diet
g. a nutrient intake value that is estimated to meet the requirement of half of the healthy individuals in a group
h. a value based on observed or experimentally determined approximations of nutrient intake by a group of healthy people

REVIEW QUESTIONS

Scenario #1: A 75-year-old patient came to the clinic with complaints of fatigue and increasing weakness. The patient had been losing weight, has a poor appetite, and noticed that their hair is dry and falls out easily.

Objective: Identify sources of dietary fiber and dietary fats.
NCLEX item type: multiple response
Cognitive skill: compare
9. The nurse reviewed the essential macronutrients needed by the body with the patient in scenario #1. Which nutrients does the nurse discuss? *(Select all that apply.)* **(772)**
   1. Fats
   2. Dietary fiber
   3. Water
   4. Proteins
   5. Carbohydrates

NCLEX item type: multiple response
Cognitive skill: classify
10. The nurse educated the patient in scenario #1 on their diet with regards to the recommended primary sources of fats. Which fat sources suggested by the nurse are considered healthy unsaturated fats? *(Select all that apply.)* **(775)**
    1. Coconut oil
    2. Olive oil
    3. Peanut oil
    4. Canola oil
    5. Soybean oil

Copyright © 2023 by Elsevier, Inc. All rights reserved.

NCLEX item type: multiple choice
Cognitive skill: contrast

11. The nurse knows that there are fat sources which have no known nutritional benefit. Which types of fats does this refer to? *(774)*
    1. Trans fats
    2. Saturated fats
    3. Polyunsaturated fats
    4. Monounsaturated fats
    5. Plant sources of fats

NCLEX item type: multiple response
Cognitive skill: analyze

12. The scenario #1 asked the nurse what was meant by dietary fiber and where it comes from. Which statements by the nurse should be included in the answer? (select all that apply.) *(778)*
    1. "A lot of the dietary fiber comes from vegetables and legumes."
    2. "There are two types of fiber; functional fiber and dietary fiber."
    3. "Dietary fiber has both indigestible and digestible carbohydrates."
    4. "Undigestible fiber has not beneficial effect."
    5. "Functional fiber may delay gastric emptying, an contributes to weight control."

Objective: Differentiate between fat-soluble and water-soluble vitamins and discuss their functions.

NCLEX item type: grid/matrix
Cognitive skill: evaluate cues

13. The nurse reviewed the types of vitamins with the patient in scenario #1. Indicate with an 'X' those vitamins that are water soluble and those that are fat soluble. *(780)*

	Water-soluble vitamin	Fat-soluble vitamin
Niacin		
Cyanocobalamin		
Retinol		
Ascorbic acid		
Biotin		
Cholecalciferol		
Phytonadione		
Pantothenic acid		
Folic acid		
Thiamine		
Alpha-Tocopherol		

NCLEX item type: multiple choice
Cognitive skill: interpret

14. The nurse was administering cholecalciferol to a patient who asks what it is. What is an appropriate response by the nurse? *(780)*
    1. "I believe this is vitamin E."
    2. "This is another name for vitamin B."
    3. "It is one of those water-soluble vitamins that are necessary in your diet."
    4. "This is vitamin D, which helps regulate calcium and phosphorus metabolism."

NCLEX item type: multiple choice
Cognitive skill: comprehension

15. The nurse discussing with a patient the foods that contain vitamin B_2 will provide further teaching after the patient makes which statement? *(780)*
    1. "Another name for vitamin B_2 is riboflavin."
    2. "I can get vitamin B_2 in my diet by eating pork, peas, and dry beans."
    3. "If I eat green leafy vegetables, fruit, and eggs, I will being getting some vitamin B_2."
    4. "I know that vitamin B_2 is important because it is needed for normal cell function."

Objective: Discuss the functions of minerals in the body.

NCLEX item type: multiple choice
Cognitive skill: explain

16. The patient with hypothyroidism asks the nurse why they can't just take iodine instead of pills for their condition. Which response by the nurse needs to be revised? *(781)*
    1. "The iodine alone would not be adequate to treat your hypothyroidism."
    2. "Iodine is just one component of the thyroid hormones you need."
    3. "You could supplement your thyroid hormones with the mineral iodine."
    4. "Dietary iodine is in seafood and dairy products and salt, but is not enough to replace your thyroid needs."

NCLEX item type: multiple response
Cognitive skill: application

17. The nurse explains to the patient in scenario #1 that there is a mineral found in grains, green leafy vegetables, nuts, and legumes that is essential for protein synthesis and nerve transmission. Which mineral will the nurse describe? *(781)*
    1. Magnesium
    2. Manganese
    3. Phosphorus
    4. Chromium

Copyright © 2023 by Elsevier, Inc. All rights reserved.

NCLEX item type: multiple choice
Cognitive skill: illustrate

18. The patient asks the nurse why minerals are important. Which statement by the nurse needs to corrected? *(781)*
    1. "Minerals such as copper is a component of enzymes needed for iron metabolism."
    2. "Calcium is an important mineral that is involved with nerve transmission, bone and teeth formation and blood clotting."
    3. "Florine found in drinking water and seafood is important for bones and teeth."
    4. "The mineral that is a component of many tissue types such as tendons and cartilage is selenium."

Objective: Describe physical changes associated with a malnourished state.

NCLEX item type: multiple response
Cognitive skill: application

19. The nurse assessed for characteristics in the patient in scenario #1 which indicates a malnourished state. What characteristics will the nurse observe for in malnourished patients? *(Select all that apply.)* *(782)*
    1. Weight loss
    2. Muscle atrophy
    3. Elevated temperature
    4. Dry hair that easily falls out
    5. Fat depletion in the waist, arms, and legs

NCLEX item type: cloze
Cognitive skill: recognize cues

Choose the most likely options for the information missing from the statements below by selecting from the list of options provided.

20. When providing patient teaching with the patient in scenario #1 regarding malnutrition, the nurse recognized the patient has _____1_____ which is characterized by _____2_____ and _____2_____. *(782)*

Option 1	Option 2
Starvation	Poor memory
Marasmus	Dry hair that falls out easily
Kwashiorkor	Intolerance of temperature changes
Mixed kwashiorkor-marasmus	Weight loss and fatigue

NCLEX item type: multiple choice
Cognitive skill: contrast

21. When patients have a protein deficiency that develops due to a diet with little or no protein but adequate fats and carbohydrates, the nurse recognizes this condition as what? *(782)*
    1. Mixed kwashiorkor-marasmus
    2. Starvation
    3. Kwashiorkor
    4. Marasmus

Scenario #2: A patient with a GI tube placed after esophageal surgery was admitted a week after discharge for tube feeding intolerance.

Objective: Describe the advantages and disadvantages of parenteral nutrition and enteral nutrition.

NCLEX item type: multiple response
Cognitive skill: application

22. What will the nurse assess when caring for the patient in scenario #2 who is on tube feedings? *(Select all that apply.)* *(787)*
    1. Checking tube placement
    2. Changing the tube feeding bag every 4 hours
    3. Monitoring for diarrhea or cramping
    4. Checking residual volumes of enteral feedings
    5. Performing daily weights and monitoring for signs of dehydration or overhydration

NCLEX item type: multiple response
Cognitive skill: analyze

23. The nurse discussed the difference between peripheral parenteral nutrition (PPN) solutions and central parenteral nutrition (CPN) solutions with a new nurse who was being oriented to parenteral nutrition. Which statements will the nurse include in the discussion? *(Select all that apply.)* *(789)*
    1. "CPN is used for patients who need nutritional support for 3 - 4 weeks; PPN is used for patients who require long-term nutritional support."
    2. "PPN solutions consist of 5% - 10% dextrose; CPN consists of 15% - 25% glucose."
    3. "CPN solutions must be administered through a central venous access line; PPN solutions may be administered through a peripheral line."
    4. "CPN solutions contain electrolytes, vitamins, and minerals; PPN solutions contain electrolytes and vitamins."
    5. "PPN solutions consist of 2% - 5% amino acids; CPN solutions consist of 3.5% - 15% amino acids."

Copyright © 2023 by Elsevier, Inc. All rights reserved.

NCLEX item type: multiple response
Cognitive skill: application
24. The nurse will monitor for which adverse effects of parenteral feedings that should be reported to the healthcare provider? *(Select all that apply.)* **(789)**
    1. Respiratory difficulty
    2. Rash, chills, and fever
    3. Hypoglycemia and/or hyperglycemia
    4. Infusion pump alarm for air in line
    5. 50 mL of solution remains in the bag after 24 hours

NCLEX item type: multiple choice
Cognitive skill: contrast
25. The nurse is discussing the advantages of enteral nutrition compared with parenteral nutrition with a patient who is going home with a gastrostomy port. Additional instruction is required after the patient made which statement? **(786)**
    1. "I know that this feeding will help stimulate my GI tract."
    2. "As you mentioned, these feedings are cheaper than if I got my nutrition in an IV"
    3. "As I understand it, there is less of a chance of infection compared with an IV."
    4. "I understand that I can use any formula since they are basically all the same."

Copyright © 2023 by Elsevier, Inc. All rights reserved.

Herbal and Dietary Supplement Therapy

chapter

47

Answer Key: Textbook page references are provided as a guide for answering these questions. A complete answer key is provided to your instructor.

MATCHING

Match the supplement on the right with its use on the left.

Use

1. _____ a common beverage used to improve cognitive performance and stimulate the CNS

2. _____ research supports that it reduces cholesterol and triglyceride levels

3. _____ used as a digestive aid for bloating, and as an antispasmodic and antiinflammatory of the GI tract

4. _____ used to alleviate nausea and vomiting from a variety of causes

5. _____ used primarily as adjunctive therapy for chronic heart failure

6. _____ used to increase the body's resistance to stress

7. _____ frequently used as a coingredient in skin care products for healing sunburn

8. _____ used for restlessness and may promote sleep

9. _____ used to reduce the frequency and severity of migraine headaches

10. _____ used to treat short-term memory loss, headaches, dizziness, tinnitus, and emotional instability

11. _____ used orally to treat mild depression and to heal wounds

12. _____ used to enhance muscle performance during exercise

Supplement

a. aloe
b. chamomile
c. creatine
d. feverfew
e. garlic
f. ginger
g. ginkgo
h. ginseng
i. green tea
j. St. John's wort
k. valerian
l. CoQ10

REVIEW QUESTIONS

Scenario #1: A 52-year-old woman came to the clinic complaining of joint pain, especially in her knees. She was told she may be getting degenerative joint disease. She told the nurse that she has been taking ginger and black cohosh.

Objective: Summarize the primary actions and potential uses of the herbal and dietary supplement products cited.

NCLEX item type: multiple choice
Cognitive skill: comprehension

13. When a diabetic patient is taking aloe, it is most important for the nurse to assess the patient for the development of which condition? *(796)*
    1. Infection
    2. Hyperglycemia
    3. Hypokalemia
    4. Hypoglycemia

NCLEX item type: multiple choice
Cognitive skill: explain

14. The nurse discusses the use of black cohosh with the patient in scenario #1, and mentions that it is contraindicated in certain patient conditions. Which statement by the nurse is correct? *(796)*
    1. "Black cohosh should not be used by patients who have arthritis conditions."
    2. "Black cohosh should not be used in the first two trimesters of pregnancy."
    3. "Black cohosh should not be used by patients who are immunocompromised."
    4. "Black cohosh should not be used by patients who are allergic to ragweed or asters."

Copyright © 2023 by Elsevier, Inc. All rights reserved.

NCLEX item type: multiple response
Cognitive skill: application

15. The nurse remarked about the common uses for chamomile and mentioned which effects it will have? *(Select all that apply.)* **(797)**
    1. Alleviate nausea and vomiting
    2. Digestive agent for bloating
    3. An antiinflammatory for skin irritation
    4. An antispasmodic for menstrual cramps
    5. A mouthwash for minor mouth irritation or gum infections

NCLEX item type: multiple choice
Cognitive skill: interpret

16. A patient with which condition is most likely to benefit from the administration of echinacea? **(797)**
    1. Multiple sclerosis
    2. Systemic lupus erythematosus
    3. Viral respiratory tract infection
    4. Acquired immunodeficiency syndrome (AIDS)

NCLEX item type: multiple response
Cognitive skill: analyze cues

17. The patient asks the nurse about the common uses for feverfew. Which conditions is feverfew found to be effect for? *(Select all that apply.)* **(798)**
    1. Alleviate nausea and vomiting
    2. Treatment of rheumatoid arthritis
    3. Reduce allergic response to ragweed
    4. Reduce the frequency and severity of migraine headaches
    5. Improve digestion and gastroesophageal reflux disease (GERD) symptoms

NCLEX item type: multiple choice
Cognitive skill: classify

18. The nurse read scientific literature that supported which common use for garlic? **(798)**
    1. Alleviate nausea and vomiting
    2. Reduce fever and inflammation
    3. Reduce cholesterol and triglycerides
    4. Improve digestion and GERD symptoms

NCLEX item type: multiple response
Cognitive skill: application

19. The patient in scenario #1 was asking the nurse what effects ginger has as an herbal preparation. Which statement would be an appropriate response from the nurse? *(Select all that apply.)* **(799)**
    1. "Ginger works as an aphrodisiac."
    2. "Ginger has no medicinal effects, so it basically works like a placebo."
    3. "Ginger has been used for centuries to alleviate nausea and vomiting."
    4. "Ginger has some modest effects in reducing the inflammation associated with rheumatoid arthritis."
    5. "Ginger has been known to reduce allergic reactions in patients with hayfever."

NCLEX item type: grid/matrix
Cognitive skill: recognize cues

20. The nurse concerned about the use of herbal medications that the patient in scenario #1 was taking, decided to look up the effects of each. Indicate with an 'X' which use or intended effect these herbal supplements have. **(799-801)**

	Ginkgo	Goldenseal	Green tea	Ginseng
Unsupported claims that it increased the body's resistance to stress				
Popular herbal medicine used to reduce inflammation of the mucous membranes				
Used primarily to increase cerebral blood flow				
Might reduce the risk of bladder, esophageal and pancreatic cancers				

Copyright © 2023 by Elsevier, Inc. All rights reserved.

Scenario #2: A patient in the outpatient clinic indicated that they were having some feelings of sadness and listlessness. The nurse reviewed their medication list and noted that the patient was taking St. John's wort. NCLEX item type: multiple response
Cognitive skill: application

21. Which statements does the nurse include when teaching the patient in scenario #2 about St. John's wort? *(Select all that apply.)* *(801)*
    1. "The active ingredients of St. John's wort are unknown."
    2. "St. John's wort is a safe drug for anyone with depression."
    3. "There are no adverse effects associated with the use of St. John's wort."
    4. "St. John's wort may cause photosensitivity, so individuals using it should avoid overexposure to the sun."
    5. "As with a lot of herbal medicines, there is no effective standardization for products such as St. John's wort"

NCLEX item type: multiple response
Cognitive skill: classify

22. The nurse reviewed the common uses for valerian and found that it is used for which effects? *(Select all that apply.)* *(802)*
    1. Laxative
    2. Sleep aid
    3. Digestive aid
    4. Alleviate restlessness
    5. Reduce inflammation

NCLEX item type: cloze
Cognitive skill: analyze cues

Choose the most likely options for the information missing from the statements below by selecting from the list of options provided.

23. The patient in scenario #2 asks the nurse what they know about CBD. The nurse responded that CBD has been researched extensively and has a variety of pharmacologic effects such as _____1_____, _____1_____, and _____1_____.
    In addition some of the adverse effects include _____2_____ and _____2_____which are important to recognize. *(802–803)*

Option 1	Option 2
Prevention of nerve degeneration	Orthostatic hypotension
Weight gain	Constipation
Antiinflammatory activity	Insomnia
Analgesia	Increased appetite

NCLEX item type: extended multiple response
Cognitive skill: recognize cues

24. The nurse knows that the provitamin coenzyme Q10 can be found in every living cell and accumulates in high levels in organs that have high energy requirements. Which organs contain the highest levels of CoQ10? *(Select all that apply.)* *(803)*
    1. Lung
    2. Brain
    3. Liver
    4. Heart
    5. Pancreas
    6. Spleen
    7. Intestines
    8. Kidneys

NCLEX item type: multiple response
Cognitive skill: application

25. A patient was explaining to the nurse why they were taking creatine. What was the most likely reason the patient is taking this supplement? *(804)*
    1. to use as a sleep aid
    2. to enhance muscle performance for short bouts of intense exercise
    3. to increase fats absorption converting it to energy
    4. to use as a weight reduction aid

NCLEX item type: multiple choice
Cognitive skill: explain

26. Why is gamma-hydroxybutyrate (GHB) available as a prescription-only product used for narcolepsy? *(805)*
    1. The adverse effects are hypertension and tachycardia.
    2. The effects of its blood-thinning properties make it too dangerous.
    3. It easily produces symptoms of nausea, vomiting, and diarrhea.
    4. It has been used as a date rape drug added to alcoholic drinks.

NCLEX item type: multiple choice
Cognitive skill: classify

27. The nurse knows there is a supplement that acts as an antioxidant and is found in tomatoes, watermelon, and pink grapefruit called what? *(805)*
    1. lycopene
    2. melatonin
    3. ginseng
    4. chamomile

NCLEX item type: multiple response
Cognitive skill: application

28. The patient in scenario #2 asks the nurse if there is a safe medication to use to help sleep. Which supplement may the nurse suggest? *(806*
    1. lycopene
    2. melatonin
    3. policosanol
    4. omega-3 fatty acids

Copyright © 2023 by Elsevier, Inc. All rights reserved.

NCLEX item type: multiple choice
Cognitive skill: explain
29. The nurse explained to a patient who asked about policosanol and what it is used for. What statement by the nurse is correct? *(806)*
    1. "Policosanol is used to decrease pulse rates."
    2. "Policosanol is used to lower blood sugar."
    3. "Policosanol is used to lower cholesterol levels."
    4. "Policosanol is used to lower blood pressure."

NCLEX item type: multiple response
Cognitive skill: illustrate
30. The nurse reviewed the plant and fish sources of omega-3 fatty acids with a patient who asked about the different foods that contain them. Which foods does the nurse mention? *(Select all that apply.)* *(807)*
    1. Tuna
    2. Sardines
    3. Soybeans
    4. Flaxseed
    5. Peanuts

NCLEX item type: multiple response
Cognitive skill: application
31. The nurse reviewed the patient conditions that are possible indications for the use of S-adenosylmethionine (SAM-e). Which conditions does the nurse recognize that SAM-e could be used for? *(Select all that apply.)* *(808)*
    1. Infection
    2. Depression
    3. Osteoarthritis
    4. Diabetes mellitus
    5. Fibromyalgia

Objective: Describe the interactions between commonly used herbal and dietary supplement products and prescription medications.
NCLEX item type: multiple choice
Cognitive skill: interpret
32. The patient in scenario #1 is on hormone replacement therapy to treat symptoms associated with menopause and to prevent osteoporosis. She also takes medication to control high blood pressure. She asks the nurse about the risks of taking black cohosh. What is the best response by the nurse? *(796)*
    1. "Black cohosh works by stimulating the body to produce its own natural testosterone."
    2. "Studies have found that black cohosh is an excellent herb for women to treat symptoms of menopause that are not controlled by hormone replacement therapy."
    3. "High blood pressure will be lowered with the use of black cohosh, so you won't need to take your high blood pressure pills any longer."
    4. "Black cohosh may cause added antihypertensive effects when taken with medication to lower blood pressure. Consult your healthcare provider before adding black cohosh to your treatment regimen."

NCLEX item type: multiple response
Cognitive skill: contrast
33. The nurse cautioned the patient taking aspirin about the herbal supplements that affect platelet aggregation and therefore should be used with caution. Which herbal supplements will the nurse discuss? *(799,800)*
    1. garlic
    2. ginseng
    3. melatonin
    4. black cohosh
    5. valerian

NCLEX item type: multiple choice
Cognitive skill: compare
34. The nurse needs to caution patients who drink alcohol or take benzodiazepines and sleep aids that the adverse effect of CNS depression may occur with the addition of which herbal product? *(806)*
    1. creatine
    2. melatonin
    3. policosanol
    4. omega-3 fatty acids

Copyright © 2023 by Elsevier, Inc. All rights reserved.

Substance Abuse

Answer Key: Textbook page references are provided as a guide for answering these questions. A complete answer key is provided to your instructor.

MATCHING

Match the slang drug name on the right with the substances of abuse on the left.

Substance of Abuse

1._____ heroin

2._____ nicotine

3._____ cocaine

4._____ marijuana

5._____ LSD

6._____ PCP

7._____ alcohol

Slang Name

a. acid

b. blow

c. booze

d. weed

e. angel dust

f. China white

g. chew

REVIEW QUESTIONS

Scenario #1: A 26-year-old woman came into the clinic for a prenatal exam and was obviously intoxicated.

Objective: Identify the differences between mild, moderate, and severe substance abuse disorder.

NCLEX item type: multiple response
Cognitive skill: application

8. The nurse reviewed the problems associated with substance abuse and knows the term *social impairment* is described as having which components? *(Select all that apply.) (811)*
   1. Craving exhibited by a powerful urge for the substance
   2. Development of withdrawal symptoms when blood levels decline
   3. Continuation of substance use in spite of persistent social problems
   4. Reduction or cessation of important social, occupational, or recreational pursuits because of substance use
   5. Failure to meet responsibilities at work, school, or home because of recurrent substance use

NCLEX item type: multiple choice
Cognitive skill: comprehension

9. The nurse reviewed the classifications for substance use disorders and when four or five symptoms are present, the patient is classified as having what? *(810)*
   1. A mild substance abuse disorder
   2. A moderate substance abuse disorder
   3. A severe substance abuse disorder
   4. A true addictive substance disorder

NCLEX item type: multiple response
Cognitive skill: application

10. The nurse recalls the symptoms included in the description of a severe substance abuse disorder. Which symptoms are part of this classification? *(Select all that apply.) (810)*
    1. A desire to cut down substance use
    2. An overwhelming compulsion to use the substance
    3. Feeling depressed when not using the substance
    4. A tolerance for higher amounts of the substance
    5. Withdrawal symptoms on discontinuation of the substance

Copyright © 2023 by Elsevier, Inc. All rights reserved.

NCLEX item type: multiple response
Cognitive skill: application

11. When providing teaching to the patient in scenario #1 about the effects of substance use and abuse with pregnancy, which statements does the nurse include? *(Select all that apply.)* **(826)**
    1. "Using alcohol and drugs while pregnant has a strong likelihood of harming the baby before and after birth."
    2. "Infants of drug addicts must be monitored closely for symptoms of withdrawal after delivery."
    3. "Using alcohol and drugs during pregnancy has a high likelihood of causing the need for induction of labor due to the fetus being postterm."
    4. "Alcohol and drug use during pregnancy has been associated with potentially fatal bleeding disorders."
    5. "Babies of mothers who used alcohol during pregnancy have a higher incidence of behavioral problems later in life."

Objective: Differentiate between the screening instruments for substance use disorders.

NCLEX item type: multiple choice
Cognitive skill: compare

12. What questionnaire will the nurse use as a quick screening instrument for assessment of alcohol abuse for the patient in scenario #1? **(814)**
    1. MMPI
    2. ADI
    3. CAGE
    4. DAST

NCLEX item type: grid/matrix
Cognitive skill: recognize cues

13. The nurse who works in the detox center realized that many of the screening instruments used for assessment of substance abuse have disadvantages. Indicate with an 'X' the advantages and disadvantages. **(814)**

	Advantage	Disadvantage
Designed as self-assessment tools		
Developed using adult male patients and have not been validated in other populations.		
Many lengthy questions not specific enough to detect the difference between excessive drinking and alcoholism		
Modified to be used as a quick-screening instrument		

	Advantage	Disadvantage
Requires an available qualified data interpreter		
Validated for accuracy used for specific purposes		

NCLEX item type: multiple response
Cognitive skill: application

14. Screening instruments used by healthcare professionals for patients who are suspected of substance abuse are divided into which four categories? *(Select all that apply.)* **(814)**
    1. Alcohol abuse screening
    2. Brief drug abuse screening
    3. Lengthy drug abuse screening
    4. Comprehensive drug abuse screening
    5. Drug and alcohol abuse screening for use with adolescents

Objective: Discuss the responsibilities of professionals who suspect substance abuse by a colleague.

NCLEX item type: multiple choice
Cognitive skill: compare

15. The nurse working with impaired patients knows that substance abuse also affects healthcare professionals. What is the incidence of abuse among this population? **(815)**
    1. Unheard of in this profession
    2. Similar to the general population
    3. Much lower than the general population
    4. Much higher than the general population

NCLEX item type: multiple choice
Cognitive skill: illustrate

16. What should a healthcare professional do if they suspect a colleague of being impaired on the job? **(815-816)**
    1. Do nothing, but keep an eye on the colleague.
    2. Confront the individual about the suspicion.
    3. Make a confidential report to the supervisor.
    4. Inform all coworkers about the situation.

NCLEX item type: multiple choice
Cognitive skill: interpret

17. A nurse was discussing their suspicions about a coworker to their supervisor and asked if the coworker was going to lose their job. What is an appropriate response by the supervisor? **(816)**
    1. "No, we cannot afford to fire anyone at this time; we are too understaffed."
    2. "Yes, but the nurse could always reapply for the job after they have been out for a year."
    3. "No, not at this point. The next step is to investigate and document any instances of impairment."
    4. "Yes, unfortunately that is the way it works. We cannot have someone impaired on the job."

Copyright © 2023 by Elsevier, Inc. All rights reserved.

Objective: Identify the withdrawal symptoms for major substances that are commonly abused.

NCLEX item type: extended multiple response

Cognitive skill: analyze cues

18. The nurse caring for a patient who was admitted with suspected opioid intoxication expects to find which signs and symptoms? *(Select all that apply.)* **(818)**
    1. Initial euphoria followed by apathy
    2. Indifference to hazardous situations
    3. Hypervigilance
    4. Increased appetite
    5. Unsteady gait
    6. Initial euphoria followed by agitation

NCLEX item type: multiple choice

Cognitive skill: classify

19. The nurse will anticipate which drug class will be used to treat alcohol withdrawal symptoms? **(819)**
    1. Adrenergic agents
    2. Benzodiazepines
    3. Cholinergic agents
    4. Anticholinergic agents

NCLEX item type: multiple response

Cognitive skill: application

20. When working with a patient who is withdrawing from long-term use of amphetamines, the nurse expects the patient to exhibit which signs/symptoms? *(Select all that apply.)* **(823)**
    1. Insomnia
    2. Fatigue
    3. Severe depression
    4. Loss of memory
    5. Inability to manipulate information

Copyright © 2023 by Elsevier, Inc. All rights reserved.